CAREGIVER
YOU ARE NOT ALONE

❧ ✾ ☙

Bobbi Carducci
the
IMPERFECT CAREGIVER

S & H Publishing, Inc.
Purcellville, Virginia

S & H Publishing, Inc.
P. O. Box 456
Purcellville, VA 20134
www.sandhpublishing.com

Publisher's Note: This work combines fiction and nonfiction. With the exception of Bobbi, her husband, Mike, and Rodger, all names, characters, places, and incidents are a product of the author's imagination. They were inspired by situations, emotions, and sentiments that, unfortunately, are very real. Any resemblance to actual people, living or dead, or to events, institutions, or locales is completely coincidental.

Ordering Information:
Quantity discounts are available. For details, contact the "Special Sales Department" at the address above or email sales@sandhpublishing.com.

Caregiver—You Are Not Alone/Bobbi Carducci
ISBN 978-1-63320-062-3 Print Edition
ISBN 978-1-63320-063-0 Ebook Edition

To my loving husband, Mike, whose support kept me whole throughout this amazing journey

INFECTED

I have already lost touch with a couple of people I used to be.
– Joan Didion

Before Rodger came to live with us, I thought I knew who I was. Up until that time I had a great track record of weathering life's challenges. When faced with hardship, I did what I had to do to solve the problem or adapted to the changes. I cried and prayed often, but never did I feel as if I'd lost myself. I didn't know I'd become infected by his illness, too.

When he wandered, I followed in his footsteps. When he lashed out at me, I lost my temper and shouted back, only to be overwhelmed with guilt once the storm had passed. When he refused to bathe for days, I'd find myself staring at my disheveled reflection in the mirror. Exhausted from lack of sleep and afraid of what he might do if I left him alone long enough to take a shower. I looked, and probably smelled, as bad as he did. Time after time we were admitted to the hospital together. Rodger to a bed, I to an uncomfortable chair beside him. We spent days and weeks together in that place.

As he continued to fail, it felt as if pieces of me were falling away. I had to face the truth. We would lose this battle.

When Rodger died, he took the person I used to be with him, and left behind a part of himself. What remained was a changed, and hopefully smarter, me. The one who writes our story. The one who would do it again for a family member if needed. The one who would not expect more from either of us than we are capable of giving.

Blessed be the caregivers both who you are now,
and who you are becoming.

❧ ❀ ☙

I was sitting at the foot of Rodger's hospital bed watching him breathe and wondering how much more he could take when he woke up and said, "I'm going back to Pittsburgh soon. There is place for me beside my wife and I am going to be with her again."

I realized he was talking about dying and a told myself not to cry. This was important, and my job in that moment was to listen. "I was dreaming and God told me my job here is done," he said. His eyes were full of wonder and I believed him. Within a few days he was admitted to in-home hospice. In the early morning hours of his eighty-third birthday, he passed away peacefully. His son was on one side of him and I was on the other, holding his hand.

Several months later, I was telling a friend of mine that I wanted to do what I could to support caregivers. I shared what Rodger had told me about his message from God and how it had touched me. "I hope you realize his job was you," my friend responded.

It had not occurred to me before that moment, but hearing it made sense. Because of the time we spent together and how much I learned from him, I am now able to do what I do to support caregivers. When he first came to live with us, I thought he would do well in my care. Little did I know that I would be trying to manage the unmanageable. I knew so little about the disease and the behavioral changes it would cause. I made mistakes that made things more difficult for both of us.

As his illness progressed, I researched Alzheimer's disease

and dementia, learning as much as I could. After his passing, I knew I wanted to share what I had learned, and do whatever I could to support caregivers. I went to caregiver conferences and workshops soaking up as much information as I could. I connected with the Alzheimer's organization and signed up for training that would allow me to become a support group facilitator and prepared me to lead a group in my local community. I completed the extensive Understanding Dementia course offered by the University of Tazmania.

In this book, I share the many things I learned. It's not a story told in a connected narrative like a novel. After all, what caregiver has time to sit and read a book cover to cover? Instead, it is told as a series of snapshots, each one complete in itself. Read it as time permits, or read it when the world closes in around you, and remember, caregivers, you are not alone.

JULIE

After Dad died I thought it was normal for Mom to be a little flaky, to forget to pay a bill or stay in her pajamas all day. She had lost the love of her life and nothing would ever be the same. I understood her grief. I wallowed in my own pain at losing Dad. It was especially hard in the quiet moments when I longed to hear his laugh or his booming voice as he sang off key with his favorite music on the car radio.

Seeing her so broken scared me. Mom was always so strong. She's the one who gathered me in her arms and got me to the hospital when I fell out of Mr. Hogan's oak tree when I was ten. Dad took one look at me, turned green and fainted. Mr. Hogan ended up taking care of him while Mom took off with me. We never told him we laughed about that on the way to the hospital.

She would find a way to get through this. It would take time but she would be herself again. Weeks later when she stopped answering the phone, I knew something was very wrong. Since the day I got married we started each day with a brief chat and and the words, "I love you."

"You never know what a day will bring and starting it off with love will get you through the rough patches when they come," she'd said.

She was right. Her love got me through a lot of bad days at work and rough patches with teenage know-it-alls. I had to be there for her now and she wasn't letting me. Determined to help her, I drove to her house, shocked to find the curtains drawn and the doors locked. Mom always loved the sun streaming in the

4

windows each morning after she fed the birds who tapped on the sliding glass doors looking for breakfast.

What I found when I finally convinced her to let me in was shocking. Clearly she hadn't bathed for several days. There were dirty dishes on the table and in the sink. The smell of sour milk was so strong I almost gagged.

"Mom, what's wrong? Are you sick? Why didn't you call me or pick up the phone when I called you?"

"Not sick, waiting, I can't do anything until he gets here."

"Until who gets here?"

"Your father. He's late. I keep waiting and he doesn't come. Sometimes I hear his car in the driveway, but he doesn't come in. Why doesn't he come in?"

"Oh, Mom. Dad can't come in. He died. Don't you remember the funeral?"

"No! He's not dead. I hear his car in the driveway. Maybe today he will come in."

That's when I knew this was more than grief and I needed to find out what was happening to her.

"Alzheimer's," her doctor said. "I've been seeing her for over a year. It probably started a few years before that."

"Oh my God. She never told me. Dad never said a word."

"She didn't want anyone to know. At first she was embarrassed, and now she doesn't know she has it. She's going to need a lot of support."

"Why didn't I notice anything before now?"

"Your father helped her hide it. He didn't like it but if that's what she wanted, he figured he's go along with her as long as he could. Losing him has brought on a huge change, and you have some very important decisions to make about her long term care. I'll admit her to the hospital for a few days. She's dehydrated and running a low grade fever. She may have a urinary tract infection. UTI's often cause changes like this in someone with Alzheimer's.

5

You take the time to talk to your husband and decide where she goes from there."

"I already know the answer to that. She's coming to live with us. Jim and I have talked about having one or more of our parents come to live with us when the day came that they needed help. We have the room and we want to do it."

"Okay, that's what we will do for now. But if it gets to be too much for you, talk to me and I'll give you information on some excellent memory care places."

"Thank you, but I don't think I'll be needing it."

"Just remember, it's here when you want it."

❧ ❀ ☙

Mom will be here in a few minutes. Jim called from the hospital to let me know when they will arrive. Are we ready for this? Any of us? Her rooms are ready, and I have plenty of her favorite food on hand. Everyone I know has someone in their family with it. Alzheimer's or dementia of some kind. Now it's got her. I'll be there for her through it all, but if it's got her now it may be coming for me or Jim later and I am scared. I hear the car pulling into the driveway. It begins.

Caregiving is a Fearsome Intimacy

When we hold our infants in our arms we are filled with awe and hope for the future. We envision a life of promises fulfilled. We never picture them feeding us, holding our hand to keep us from falling, or changing our underthings. I don't even like to type the word *diapers*. The thought of losing one's dignity to such a degree is truly fearsome. In my mind I hear the words, "It's enough to scare the pants off me." The irony makes me shudder and chuckle at the same time.

The caregiver and the cared for locked in a fearsome

6

intimacy. I don't know where the quote came from. If I did, I would give credit here. What I do know is those five simple words speak a devastating truth.

BETH

Bill had another stroke. His third, and the doctor said he'd had several TIAs (Transient Ischemic Attacks) before this one hit. I am so mad I could spit. How many times was he advised to lose weight and stop smoking over the years? Dozens? Hundreds?

Then he was diagnosed with sleep apnea. He stopped breathing several times a minute, for Pete's sake. He could have died in his sleep right next to me. I don't even want to imagine what that would have been like. He was given a C-PAP machine to keep his airway open when he sleeps. It's ugly and awkward but it keeps him alive and it's a whole lot quieter than that terrible snoring that used to drive me out of our room most nights. Hell, I could still hear him from downstairs. He was told he would probably start dreaming again since he would finally be getting some REM sleep. It worked. In fact it worked so well I started dreaming again too. I guess all that snoring had an effect on me as well. I told him that I read in one of the pamphlets that came with his machine that if he got within ten percent of normal weight he probably wouldn't have sleep apnea anymore. Did that get him to lose weight? No, it didn't.

Then he got Type II diabetes. Of course he was told to lose weight and limit his carbohydrate intake. He didn't have to avoid them altogether. A balanced meal on his plate would be half vegetables, one quarter protein, and one quarter carbohydrates. That makes sense to me. Did he do it? No, of course not.

Through it all I prayed. "God, give me strength. Let me be patient with him. Food is everywhere and changing is hard."

The first stroke was a mild one. A warning his doctor told him. "Do something to change your diet or you're asking for another one."

He took the blood thinners, dieted for a few weeks and went right back to his old habits.

I prayed for strength to help him get back on track and to stifle the resentment that he was risking my life along with his. I love him and need him in my life; why can't he understand that?

Stroke number two was another warning. He got to the hospital in time for a clot buster to save him. He wasn't so lucky with number three. This time the doctor said there is brain damage from the stroke and the TIAs.

"He's going to have some cognitive impairment; how severe we don't know yet."

Three weeks in, we have a better idea. His short term memory is gone. He's mean as a snake at times and he keeps saying he wants a divorce. A few minutes later he's telling me how much he loves me. He wants to run away and get married. That would be sweet except he calls me Marla and goes on and on about my gorgeous blond hair. That's hard for this true brunette to deal with.

Our son came over and installed hand rails and a handicapped toilet in the bathroom. Bill's legs are weak and he's a fall risk. He hates his walker and only uses it when he knows I'm watching him. He's going to take a hard fall one of these days, I know it. Then I will really need strength. He can't eat as much as he used to, that would be a good thing to come out of this, except he keeps accusing me of starving him and threatening to call the police. So each night I pray. God, are you listening? Please grant me strength to go on.

Be Careful What You Pray For

Please God, grant me strength."
I have said those words many times. Like most people I have experienced love and loss, joy and pain, happiness and grief. During the good times I pray to say thank you for my blessings and to ask God's protection for my loved ones. I pray for peace. Quite often I pray for things I want. (I'm no saint, after all.)

During the hard times I used to pray for the strength to see me through. I knew no matter how hard things became there would be an end to my suffering. I just needed to be strong enough to see it through. When I lost a baby via miscarriage, I paced and prayed well into the night until exhaustion finally overtook me. I prayed so long, so hard, when my sister died I barely slept for weeks. As a single mother of four I dealt with the many challenges with hope and prayer every day.

Despite my almost constant request for strength my prayers never seemed to be answered. Instead of giving up I prayed more and I prayed harder. After all, God is busy and it often takes time for our prayers to be answered. I dug in and did my best to get through each crisis, and when it was over, I'd pray for the strength to get through the next one. I always knew more trouble would follow.

Then one day, as I was sharing my woes with a friend, I ended my tale with the same words I so often repeated. "God, grant me strength."

"Oh, Honey,don't say that," she said. "Look what you've been through. What you've survived. You're strong enough already, don't you think?"

"I know I'm strong but I never know what I'll have to deal with next. I have to make sure I'm ready for whatever comes my way."

"That may be true, but the last thing you need is to become stronger. Think about what you have to do to get strong. If you want to build muscle you lift heavy weights. The stronger you want to become the heavier weight you have to lift and the more often you have to heft it. Is that what you want?"

"No. I want the burden to be lifted. I want help. I want to know how to solve the problem before it becomes too much for me."

"Then that's what you should ask for. Don't forget that God endowed us with an intellect and free will. We are in charge of our lives. He assists us when asked but he doesn't take over and fix our problems. He provides us with opportunities to work them out in our own way. When you ask for strength he provides you with opportunities to become strong. If you ask for patience you will be given opportunities to learn how to wait. Be careful what you pray for. Consider what you really need and ask for that."

"What do you mean?"

"If you need help, ask for help. If you are lost, ask Him to show you the way. Whatever you do stop asking for strength.

I thought about her advice for a long time. It made sense and it wouldn't hurt to change the words to my nightly prayers. I stopped asking for strength. Years later, after I had been a caregiver for a long time and things were especially hard, I prayed almost constantly for weeks.

"Please send help. Dear God, I need help. Please send help any way you see fit." Despite my prayers, Rodger ended up in the hospital again. Still I prayed. Even on the way to sit at his bedside and feed him, I prayed. "I need help. Show me the path you want me to take."

When I arrived at his room, a man was standing at the door waiting for me. "Mrs. Carducci, do you need help?" he said.

Not sure I'd heard him right, I asked him to repeat what he'd said.

"I see in Rodger's files that you've been caring for him for a long time and his needs are extensive. Do you need help?"

After taking the time to say a silent prayer of thanks in recognition to God for answering my prayers, I assured the man I did, indeed, need help. Before I left the hospital that day, we were enrolled in a respite program that would mean I would have in-home help eight hours a week. I could finally get some rest. I could go to the grocery store. I could go to church and say a proper thank you.

Each night when I say my prayers, I ask God to hold me in His love and light and show me the path He wants me to take. The road is often long and bumpy but I always end up where I need to be, and I am grateful. I have no need to become stronger.

CHARLIE

O f course you're too damned busy to give me a break! When are you not? I never thought I'd have to do this alone. When Dad got sick and we held that family meeting, you promised to help. It made sense for me to be the one to take him in. I was retired and could stay home and take care of him.

Take care of him. That sounds so strange, even after three years of doing it. Who would have thought that any of us would ever have to take care of Dad? The bigger than life, stronger than Paul Bunyan, guy who worked from sunup to sundown six days a week and half days on Sunday? I don't know about you, but I thought he was invincible.

I remember the day Jack Peters had that car accident. He was thrown out through the unlocked door and the car rolled over on his leg trapping him in agony. Dad was coming home from the feed store and he saw Jack's car crumpled in the middle of the road. Somehow he managed to pick up the front end and pull Jack out from under it. He used his own belt as a tourniquet to stop the bleeding, carried Jack to his truck and got him to the hospital in time for the surgeon to save his leg. When people started calling Dad a hero, he'd have none of it.

"I just did what anyone would do. You see a guy lying in the road you can't just drive by and leave him there. Wouldn't be right."

That's what I feel you are doing. You see Dad, how he is now, and me, wearing out caring for him, and you drive on by. You promised to help. You know you did. And when I ask you to come and stay for a day or two so I can get some rest, you always have an excuse why you can't this time. This time, really? What time did you do it? "Oh, not now, but next time." Yes, that's always it, isn't it?

If you can't help me, can you at least call or visit him more than once or twice a year? He asks about you, you know. He even brags about how busy and important you are. I wonder how he'd feel if he knew how selfish you are. How you take your family on vacations and how you simply don't have time to visit him or call him other than on his birthday or a holiday.

He's failing. I don't know how much longer he'll be here. His heart's getting weaker. He can't bathe or dress himself anymore. I feed him his meals. He looks so small now. Every day he seems more diminished and every day takes a toll on me.

No one can go without a good night's sleep indefinitely. But for some reason you seem to believe I can. Why am I all alone in this?

Brother Where Art Thou?

Questions Caregivers Long to Ask:

- ➢ Why aren't you here more often?
- ➢ What gives you the right to question and demand answers about how diminished he's become when you only come by once or twice a year?
- ➢ Why don't you call once week or even once a month if you're concerned?
- ➢ What? You're leaving on vacation and will be gone for three weeks? I haven't had a vacation, or even a day off, in five years. Hell, an hour to myself would be a treat.
- ➢ How is he? What do you mean, how is he? He's

sick. He has dementia and Parkinson's disease. He can't swallow anything but pureed food. He forgets where he is. He forgets who we are. He's failing fast. You should stop by and see him before you go away. Will you?

➤ You have too much to do to get ready for your trip? You'll call when you get back? If he needs anything while you're gone can I give you a call on your cell phone?"

➤ And if I call, what will you do? Will you interrupt your trip? Will you come home early to care for him? We both know the answer to that. You already paid for the hotel. There will be a big fee for changing your airline tickets. It doesn't make sense to rush back when there is nothing you can do for him.

➤ Nothing you can do for him or nothing you choose to do for him? Where are you when he misses you? Where are you when he's in the hospital again? Where are you when he's tired of dealing with me, and we both need a break?

➤ Where are you in the middle of the night when he sets off the bed alarm—every few minutes—all night long?

➤ Where are you when the sun goes down and he gets combative?

➤ Where you are when the doctor asks if there is anyone else to help care for him because it's clear the stress is taking a huge toll my health?

➤ Brother where art thou, and where will you be when I can't do this anymore?

KATE

I saw Sue in the grocery store today. I tried to swerve into the closest aisle so she wouldn't see me. I know I look a mess, but I had to get in and out of there while John's favorite show was still on. For some reason he freaks out if he misses a rerun of that old western show, *Bonanza*.

Sue looked so nice in her cute outfit. Her hair and makeup just right as always. I used to look like that. Now I run out of the house in a pajama top and a pair of jeans I've worn for three days. This face hasn't had makeup on it in months. She spotted me before I could get away and was kind enough not to mention my disheveled appearance. She asked about John. She wanted to know if he's improving. I wanted to scream. I hear that question so often. Why don't people understand that with what he has he will never get better? He's slowly dying. Piece after piece of him is being stolen by this horrible disease called Lewy-Body dementia. I can hardly breathe sometimes I'm so sacred.

"Let me know if I can do anything to help," she said.

I wish I knew what to say to that. The need is so great I don't know where to start.

A Caregiver Near You Needs Help

"There are only four kinds of people in this world: those who have been caregivers, those

16

who are currently caregivers, those who will be caregivers and those who will need caregivers."
— *Former First Lady Rosalyn Carter*

According to the Caregiver Action Network there are over 65,000,000 people caring for family members in the United States at any given time. Most caregivers are women, and they need our help.

They may not say it out loud but they *are* communicating their need in their absence from all the activities in which they used to be involved. It's evident by the phone calls, text messages and tweets that no longer arrive in your inbox. Perhaps the last time you saw this caregiver in the grocery store there was a brief moment when he or she was fighting back tears.

Maybe you asked what you could do to help and were told everything was fine. Yet, as she walked away, somewhere inside, you knew it wasn't true.

You may have offered to help many times only to be thanked politely for the thought and never taken up on your offer. Some of you may have started to wonder if she really wants help.

"Why should I keep offering if that's the way it's going to be?" you may have asked yourself.

The answer is, "Because she needs help. She wants help. If she doesn't get help she is going to break under the pressure." Often she doesn't know what to ask for.

How do you request a good night's sleep or a few moments to collect your thoughts?

How do you tell friends who are so busy with their own families that you are lonely and wish they would stop by for a visit now and then?

How do ask someone to keep you from falling when every moment of your time is spent holding on for dear life to another?

17

Somewhere a caregiver is trying hard to hold it all together.

If you know a caregiver, please don't ask if she needs help. Know that she does.

ANN

"Mom, open your eyes one more time, please." I've read that people who are unresponsive can hear what we say to them. I hope it's true.

It would be such a gift to have her awake one more time. I want to let her know I'm sorry for the times I was angry and resentful when taking care of her took over my life. There's a saying that a person with dementia isn't giving you hard time; the person with dementia is having a hard time. Well guess what? It's both.

You were having a hard time and giving me one too. I tried to remember it was the disease talking when you called me a no good bitch, or when you threw your dinner plate at me. What possessed you to hide your soiled underwear in your closet? I still can't figure that out. What were you saving it for? When the smell got bad, you accused me of poisoning your air. When I finally realized where it was coming from I really lost it. I called you a crazy old bat. I'm so sorry, Mom.

I hope you know I would never steal from you. Your money is still in your bank account, every penny of it. I wish you could walk out of here and see that for yourself. The first time you accused me I felt so betrayed. I don't want your money. I'd give you everything I have if it would help you to get better.

I don't want to remember you this way. Open your eyes, please. I'm praying for one more moment when I am your child and not your caregiver. I don't like where real life has taken us. I'll be your little girl again if that's the only way you will recognize me. We can play pretend and fill a little teapot with water and

19

serve it in tiny cups. You can show me again how to take the crust off peanut butter and jelly sandwiches and cut them into quarters. We'll lift our pinkie finger when we sip our tea and dab our mouth with paper napkins we decorated with crayons. I still have one of those napkins. Can you believe I saved it all these years?

Where are you now, Mom? Are you absorbing all the mysteries of the universe? Are angels whispering to you about what's waiting for you on the other side? I hope that in this moment you are in a place that brings you joy.

Reality – What Is It Good For?

Get real. Get your head out of the clouds.
Stop daydreaming and get to work.

How many times in your life have you heard or said those words? I heard them a lot. I loved lying on my back in a field of sweet smelling grass as fluffy summer clouds turned into magical beings right before my eyes. Sometimes, I'd spot or horse or an elephant. Once I saw an image of my math teacher reaching for a hot dog. I laughed so hard my sides hurt. As a writer, I know the value of pushing reality aside to explore a world of possibilities. As a caregiver; I found that letting go of reality sometimes opened a rare portal to communication.

One of my favorite memories of my mother is when she and I took an amazing trip far from the real world and connected in a way I will always treasure.

I'd come from Virginia, lugging my suitcase and my fears to care for her. She was finally resting after a twenty-four hour marathon conversation with the universe. Rambling on incoherently at times, speaking

20

clearly at others, she took me on an unforgettable adventure of fantasy and memory.

"Wow, look at that!" she said. Her eyes wide with wonder.

"I see," I tell her.

"What is it?"

Uh oh. What do I say now?

"What is it?" she asked again, this time a fearful note in her voice.

"I don't know, what do you think it is?" I answered.

"I think it's a bee. I hope it doesn't sting me."

"I won't let it get you. I'll swat it if it comes close again."

"Okay." She sighed, relieved to know that she was no longer in danger.

"Do you have to go on tonight?"

Go on? Go on what? I thought.

"I don't think so," I told her. "I'll have to check my schedule."

"I never knew you could sing. When did you learn to sing like that?"

Sing? Me? No way. I laughed to myself. I'm the one they couldn't decide where to place in the second grade choir because the director couldn't figure out if I was an alto or a soprano. My voice is *that* bad. I was pleased that she gave me a talent I always wanted. I wondered if she could also make me a real blonde. Fix it so I no longer have to spend hours at the hairdresser to look more like my beautiful sister.

"Sing to me. Sing me a song so I can rest."

So I sang.

"You are my sunshine, my only sunshine. You make me happy when skies are grey..."

The visiting nurse raised her eyebrows and covered her ears. I shrugged my shoulders in a "What're ya

21

gonna do" gesture and continued singing. Mom relaxed in my arms.

"Sleep tight," I whispered, only to see her eyes pop open, once again.

"Look, look over there," she said, pointing. "I see angels. Three of them, right over there. They have light all around them but I don't see any wings."

"Yes, I see them." I placated her. "They've come to watch over you as you sleep. Get some rest now." I began again. "You are my sunshine......"

"Oh, please." She rolled her eyes. "Stop that racket if you expect me to get any sleep. Who do you think you are, some lounge singer?"

Smiling, I watched as she drifted into sleep, thankful for the gift of song, even if we shared it only for a little while.

We were up and down all night long; I saw her chasing shooting stars, crying over a ruined party dress, livid with rage for some unknown man from her past. I saw the wonder in her eyes as she held her firstborn child. Laughed as she went skinny dipping with my Dad in the creek behind their first house. For a time she spoke a language no one else could define, growing frustrated with my lack of understanding until she looked at me and said, "I love you." I can recognize that in any language. Finally, seeing I understood, she drifted into a deep peaceful sleep that lasted for hours. When she awoke she was back to reality, an old woman weakened by non-Hodgkin's lymphoma and chemotherapy. Gone were the angels and the memories of a life full of possibilities. Tears filled my eyes as I bathed her and prepared for the day ahead. Reality, who needs it?" I said softly, and looked forward to the evening to come.

Unless your loved ones are combative or a danger to

themselves or others it's best to go with them wherever their memories take them. Their sense of time and place is as real to them as yours is to you and trying to convince them otherwise just adds to your stress and theirs. And who knows, you may end up with a talent you always wish you had.

PETER

"Hey good looking." My wife batted her eyes at me and smiled. "Come here often?"

"Every day, Toots. How about you?"

"That's for me to know and you to find out. Are you going to the dance tonight?"

"I am if you'll be there. Will you save a few dances for me?"

"That depends."

"On what?"

"How well you dance. I don't need you stepping all over my feet all night."

"None of the other girls have complained, so I guess I do all right."

"So you're one of those guys, huh?"

"What guys?"

"The ones that flirt with all the girls."

"Not anymore."

"What's that supposed to mean?"

"It means that after seeing you, I don't want to dance with the other girls anymore."

"Sure, I'll bet that line works pretty good for you."

"Never tried it. It's not a line. So will you go to the dance with me?"

"I tell you what. I'll go to the dance. If you happen to be there, I'll save a waltz for you. And you better not step all over my feet."

❧ ✳ ☙

"Oh, hello, Mr. Carter. I didn't know you were here," the day

24

nurse said entering the room. "Are you going dancing tonight?"

"Yes, we are. I love it when she remembers our first date."

"I think she does, too. Who wouldn't want to be young and falling in love again? I'm glad you're smart enough to go there with her."

"I wouldn't miss it for anything. I get to be a young man holding the most beautiful girl in the world in my arms again. That's a moment I hope neither of us ever forgets."

Cherish The Moment

I live in my own world, but it is okay. They know me here.

—Author Unknown

If today our loved ones are young again, running barefoot with the wind rippling through their hair, join them in their moments of freedom. It is far easier for us to enter their world than for them to enter ours.

If your mother or father doesn't recognize you today, it may be because in his or her mind they are still becoming the person who will hold you in the future. It doesn't take away a single moment of the time the two of you shared. You are the memory keeper as they relive the moments that came before. Each of you have a gift to share with the other. Cherish the moment.

KELLY

My friend at work told me her mother has Alzheimer's. My grandmother has it. I know a lot of people get it when they get old. But I didn't know someone could forget their own child. I can see how you can forget where you put your car keys or to pay your bills on time. But to not remember a kid you gave birth to; that's crazy. And Laurie is thirty years old. It's not as if the woman just had a baby and got sick. Laurie and her mom were like best friends. They used to go shopping together. They went to the movies all the time; they even look alike.

I wonder if Grammie will forget my mom or me. The last time I went to see her, she called me Patty. She thought I was her sister. Aunt Pat is old. How can she get us mixed up like that? She tried to laugh it off when I told her who I was, but she looked kind of scared. I didn't think it was funny either. Alzheimer's is some weird shit. I hope my mother doesn't get it.

She Doesn't Remember Me

Four of the saddest words ever spoken.
I hope my children never have a reason to say them. But it could happen. If it does, I hope they know that even in my confused mind they are still in there with me.

By the time I reach that point I will have lost much already:

My short term memory.

My rich vocabulary.

My love of long, hot showers.

My ability to cook.

My driver's license or even how to find my way home if I did still have that privilege.

I pray I'll still have the ability to read and understand the words my favorite authors have so painstakingly crafted. A world without books would be barren indeed for someone who loves to read as much as I do.

Alzheimer's or some other form of dementia will have taken me somewhere back in time. Perhaps I am reliving my days as a busy young mother and you, my darling daughter or son, are still in elementary school. You have not yet grown into the wonderful adult you will become. I see you pink cheeked and out of breath after running up the steps, opening the screen door, and calling out, "Mom, I'm home. Guess what I got on my spelling test today!"

It may not seem like it in the moment, but the memory of you is deeply implanted in my heart. The heart that beat so close to yours during the time I carried you. The heart that cried with you when you were hurt and rejoiced with you when you achieved a goal.

If the day comes when I look at you and ask, "Who are you?" I hope you will smile and tell me your name and share memories of your mother.

I love you. I pray you never forget that.

LESLIE

What the hell is wrong with you people? I'm here every single God damned day and you have the nerve to come in here and question me? Where are you when she wants to know where her keys are every two seconds? She hasn't had a need for keys in five years, but she demands I give her the keys to the boxes. I have no idea what boxes she is talking about. She probably doesn't either. I gave her an old key one day, hoping it would end the incessant demands. It did for a while. The peace and quiet was wonderful. Then I walked into the room and realized she was using the key to rip holes in her leather chair. When I took it from her, she screamed at me, and threatened to call the cops on me for holding her hostage.

I know she seems fine to you. The big faker. I don't know how she does it. She can be confused and combative for hours, swearing a blue streak at the people on the television or at me for some imagined slight, and as soon as you come in, she's coherent and almost normal. You don't see what I see. You don't live with this every day. You know she's sick. Why don't you believe me when I tell you what this is like?

You should come and stay with her for a few days and see for yourself! I'd love to hear what you'd have to say after that. Unless you live with this, there's no way you can understand. You have no right to judge me. If you only knew what I'd like to say to you.

A Much Nicer Way to Say It

Open your mouth only if what you are going to say
is more beautiful than silence.   —*Arabic Proverb*

Shut...the...hell...up! That's what caregivers would like to say. No, not say, scream, when family members drop by for a short visit and begin to offer comments like this:

"She looks fine to me. Why do you pretend taking care of her is harder than it is?"

"Mom told me her things are disappearing. What's going on?"

"What do you mean it's time to look at placing Dad in a nursing home? I promised him I'd never do that."

"He's lost a lot of weight. Why aren't you feeding him enough?"

"I can't take her. I have a very busy life. You get to stay home all day and watch TV."

"I should have known better than to invite you! You always have some lame excuse."

"We can't make it for his birthday. We're leaving for vacation in Italy that day."

Instead of telling them to shut up we cringe, bite our tongue, and fume in silence all too often. It would be nice to cut loose with how we really feel, but we don't. I wonder why that is?

One day I was thoroughly fed up with the bullshit and decided to stop taking it. At the same time I didn't want to make things worse for me. I didn't care if they were stressed. In fact I hoped they would be. Fair is fair after all.

I struggled to find a way to respond that would get my point across and let them know how I really felt in a way that would hit them later, after the visit was over.

29

Bobbi Carducci

Eventually I came up with this. "I hear what you are saying and I'll give your comments all the consideration they deserve. Bless your heart."

If you're from the south you will appreciate the last three words I uttered.

30

JAMES

I thought I could do this. I thought I knew what kind of man I am. Now, I know only one thing: I don't know what the hell I am doing. I can't believe I lost it like that. I know he's sick. He can't help being like this. He would be so embarrassed if he realized what has happened to him.

Why do I let his behavior get to me? I am failing him. If I can't figure this out he's going to continue to get worse. He is getting worse. I'm getting worse along with him.

As hard as I try, I can't get past the belief that sometimes he does things on purpose to get to me. He used to do that with Mom. He'd deliberately do something to set her off and then go for a walk. He never would admit it, but he'd wink at me as he went out the door. I think he's in there somewhere doing the same thing to me. And I fall for it.

If I were smarter, more patient, a better man, he might not be so hard to deal with. If I could control my feelings better this would be easier. I don't like who I am sometimes. It's no wonder he doesn't either.

Do Not Believe the Things You Tell Yourself

I know the voice of doubt. It comes in the night to question and criticize. It tells us we are not good enough or smart enough to do this. It may come as a whisper or scream unceasingly. Either way, it keeps us awake going over the activities of the day.

"Why do you keep asking if she remembers?

"How could you lose your temper? You know he's sick."

"I can't believe you said that to him."

"How could you forget to tell the doctor about that?"

"You think you're so smart, why is she getting worse every day?

Yes, I know the voice of doubt. I know how we question ourselves all the time. We expect so much of ourselves it's impossible to live up to our expectations. When family members question us, we get angry. When we do it to ourselves, we start to believe. We lose precious sleep judging ourselves harshly.

I know the voice of doubt. She whispered to me every night. She lied. I hope by writing this, I will be able to convince you that the voice keeping you awake at night is no better than mine was. You are a caregiver, and you do not have to be perfect to do what is best for the person in your care. Forgive yourself.

THOMAS

I called my brother again today. He didn't pick up—as unusual. He knows why I'm calling. He hasn't been here since Dad's last birthday. In a week it will be here again. Dad pretends it doesn't bother him, but I know better. He keeps asking, "When will Dan come?" When I tell him I don't know, he tries to shrug it off, but I see the pain in his eyes. It's the same with his own brother. A ten minute visit every six months or so and he's gone. The last time Dad cried. He tried to convince me his eyes were watering from allergies. He doesn't have allergies, but I let him think I bought it. There's no sense in arguing. He will always find a way to make sure his brother is not at fault for anything.

I know better. His excuse is that it's too hard to see Dad this way. "If you knew him when he was a young man in Italy, so strong he could work in the fields for hours without stopping. He carried twice as many crates of grapes to the winepress as any other man each year and still had enough energy left to dance with all the pretty girls on Saturday night. He was smart too. A genius in some ways. He did calculus in his head and loved learning new languages. It breaks my heart to see him this way."

It breaks my heart too. I see him every day. I know what he has lost and what he will continue to lose. The fact that he is so diminished is exactly why you should be here for him now. He needs the connection to the past that your presence brings. He lives there most of the time now, in his long term memories. With you, he can be that vital young man again. Shame on you for denying him that.

It's Too Hard to See Him Like That

Caregivers, how often do you hear those words from family members trying to justify avoiding your loved one? For refusing to help even long enough to give you a few hours or days of respite? They may feel that we will understand that they would like to help but they simply can't.

We know what they are really saying is:

"It's too hard and it doesn't matter how it affects anyone else. It's not about Mom or Dad. It's not about our brother or sister. It's about me and how I feel."

"Mom doesn't know me anymore so why bother visiting? When I do come by, all she does is repeat the same stories over and over. It's boring and irritating. I can't take it.

I feel that way sometimes too. That's why I need your help. Why can't you understand that?"

"She was up all night for the past two weeks and you desperately need sleep? Take a nap during the day when she does. What's your problem?"

"It's not safe. If she wakes before I do, she could leave the house and wander away. She could decide to cook something and forget it on the stove and start a fire."

"He's combative and accuses you of stealing from him? What did you do to set him off? What do expect me to do about it?"

"I didn't set him off. The disease did. I don't expect you to fix it. I need you to understand what's happening."

She seemed fine to me the last time I visited."

If that's true why don't you come more often? Why are you too busy to give me a break?

"My father would never use language like that! Why would you say such things about him? I think you're the one who has a problem."

Yes, I have a problem. It's trying to deal with all this and you, too. Would you like me to tape record him for you?

"A nursing home? Never! I promised Mom we would never do that to her."

"We also promised to take care of her. When did "we" become only me?"

"If things are so bad, put her in a nursing home. What do you mean you need help to pay for it? What about her social security and Medicare?"

The facilities that would take her for what little she receives are full with long waiting lists. You clearly haven't seen what goes on in those places. One of us would have to be there every day to make sure she gets the care she needs, and we know who that would be."

ELLEN

I wish people would stop telling me what to do and how to do it. Maybe their mother, brother, sister, or friend did have dementia. Maybe they saw a documentary about it on television, but that does not make them an expert on how to live with someone you love whose brain is being eaten away a little bit at a time.

I want them to stop assuring me everything will be okay! It won't. Perhaps the medicine someone's sister's best friend's mother took did help. I'm sure it did for a while. But for how long? How much good did it do?

Have I tried being more patient? Yes. I try every day and sometimes I can do it. I'm ashamed to say that sometimes I can't.

He needs to get out more? He can't walk anymore and he refuses to sit in the wheelchair. He's incontinent and rips off his pants when he pees in them. Sometimes he takes his pants down and pees on the floor so they don't get wet. Are you going to take him out?

Most people mean well, but far too many don't know what they are talking about. They don't live this. I do.

Get the Hell Off My Mountain

There are hundreds of paths up the mountain, all leading in the same direction, so it doesn't matter which path you take. The only one wasting time is the one who runs around and around the mountain, telling everyone that his or her path is wrong. *–Hindu Proverb*

Just as there are many paths up the mountain there are many paths of caregiving. How ours will twist and turn depends on the reason it began in the first place and how the one in our care responds to the many obstacles in the way. Will he reach for me to help guide him along the way, or will he insist on refusing my assistance, only to fall and accuse me of pushing him?

Every day, around each new bend, we are faced with something unexpected. It could be a breathtaking moment when the sun breaks through the clouds of confusion and he smiles. I feared I'd never see that twinkle again. "Thank you, Lord."

Far more likely it's another loss making every step we take together more difficult. Our path is longer and far more difficult that we could have imagined. It is, also, the way that works for us. We figure it out as we go along.

The last thing we need is "the one who runs around the mountain, telling everyone that his or her path is wrong."

Unfortunately, there seems to be as many of them as there are of us. If you are dealing with someone like that, send them this Hindu proverb. And tell them the Imperfect Caregiver says, "You are not helping. You are making things more difficult."

GET THE HELL OFF THE MOUNTAIN.

JOY

Sometimes you have to laugh or you will start to cry and not be able to stop. Yesterday was like that for me. Mom refused to take a shower, again. She wouldn't even wash her face for me. It's been over a week. She's beginning to smell bad. Rather than argue and get her in a tizzy, I decided to let it go and try again later.

I got dressed myself and decided that while she was resting I'd do some laundry. I took her hamper from her room and carried it downstairs. Imagine my surprise when I found her dentures in there. She had her teeth in when I was trying to get her to shower. She must have put them in the hamper while I was in my room. I have to wonder why she thought her teeth belonged in the hamper, but I don't expect I'll ever know. Perhaps she was hiding them for some reason or maybe she thought they needed to be cleaned. I set them aside to return to her when she was in a better mood and got on with my task.

I picked up the empty pill sorter I'd placed on the counter to remind me to order refills for the month. I don't know when she had gotten into that, but when I opened the tab for Wednesday, I found four olive pits nestled in there. Fortunately, the sorter with her medication in it was safely locked up in my room. I shook my head, tossed the pits in the trash, and finished the laundry.

Hearing her talking to herself, I entered her room and suggested, again, that she take a shower. She was even more adamant that time. No shower. Again, I let it go. Tomorrow would be another day, and one has to pick ones battles, or go insane trying to reason with her.

If only someone could keep an eye on her for a while. I would love a long hot shower to ease the tension out of my shoulders. And a luxurious shampoo, taking the time to lather, rinse, and repeat like it says on the bottle. After drying off, I'd put sweet smelling lotion all over me, slip into a silk nighty, and go to sleep. Right, that's about as likely to happen as Mom deciding to do the same. Sigh. I wonder what she's up to now.

Give a Caregiver a Bath

When my husband and I first announced we were bringing his ill father to live with us, many well-meaning people assured us they would be there to help when needed, and they meant it. I remember saying, "We are going to need some time off once in a while so we can go on vacation or out to dinner. It will be great if I can call on you then."

"Of course," was the answer, and they meant it.

I didn't know then that going out to dinner or taking a vacation would not be what I would come to need most. As my father-in-law's illnesses progressed, what I longed for was an hour to take a long hot shower or to soak in tub of water up to my chin until my fingers and toes turned pruney. I'd have done just about anything to stop listening for signs he was in distress or that he somehow knew I wasn't paying attention and had decided to go down the stairs unattended, risking a fall. Even an uninterrupted ten minutes in the bathroom would have been a gift on some days.

One morning in particular, he'd had his breakfast and I had helped him wash and dress. I'd seen to it that he had his medications, and the TV was tuned to his favorite show. He should have been good for at least thirty minutes. About to start a load of laundry, I felt the sudden urge to pee. I had just settled on the toilet, when I heard him calling.

"Bobbi! Bobbi! Come quick, I need you!"

He sounded so frantic I was afraid of what I would discover when I got to him. I jumped up in mid-stream, pulled my pants up, and ran up the stairs.

"What's wrong?" I asked, ignoring the warmth running down my leg.

"The TV's gone berserk. I can't get any channels."

I bit my tongue, fixed the TV, and went to my room for a quick wash up and change of clothes. Clearly it was going to be one of those days.

If anyone had asked what I needed that day, the answer would have been easy: "I need a bath."

LEN

I don't know if I can do this. I hate to admit it, but I'm terrified. I didn't think I'd ever say that, but I am. If anyone tried to harm her physically, I'd have no problem jumping in to save her. I don't care how big the person might be or how many people were threatening her, I'd fight to the death to save her if need be. But this? I have no weapons or special skills that can save her. There are none. That's what the doctors tell me. How many are treating her now? Four or is it five?

Primary doctor, cardiologist, psychiatrist, dementia specialist, and the neurologist. That's right, five of them. And a visit with one or more of them twice a month. A total of eighteen pills a day. Nothing changes despite all the medication. She will never get better. She will definitely get worse. No cure. No hope. No timeline. It's cruel and unusual punishment for both of us, and we have done no great wrong, committed no crime or unforgiveable sin.

The raw truth is that I am already mourning her. Losing her while she is here is an agony far greater than I ever thought possible to endure. Yet it continues and the pain grows more with each loss she faces. I am terrified of what tomorrow will bring.

Caring Takes Courage

Courage doesn't always roar. Sometimes courage is the little voice at the end of the day that says I'll try again tomorrow.

—*Mary Anne Radmacher*

Caring takes courage. The courage to open your home and heart to what is to come. The courage to advocate fiercely for those in your care. The courage to know the day may come when you will hear the words, "Who are you?" from your mother or father.

Sometimes it takes every ounce of your brave spirit to get up and face another day. Yet you do. You continue even when you feel a desperate need to run away from it all.

There may be days when you do roar. When you rage against these terrible diseases. When you fight with your spouse over the unfairness of it all, or in dark moments, when you lose your temper with the one in your care. Yes, it will happen to you, and it happens to others.

It happened to me. When it did, I cowered in shame, appalled at what I perceived as weakness. When had I become less than I once was? Nothing but a coward, afraid of what another day would bring. I cried. I prayed. I vented. And I cried some more.

Finally, as the tears fell, washing away some of the stress and my strength grew, I remembered those three powerful words, *Caring Takes Courage*. Then reassured, I slept, and regained the courage to try again tomorrow.

AMY

There are not enough hours in the day to get things done. Cook, clean, pack lunches for school, get the big kids off in the morning. Why can't they get up when their alarm goes off? Why do I have to call them at least five times before they stumble out of bed, grouchy as all get out? I still have to help the two younger ones get dressed, eat some cereal, and brush their teeth. Wait with them for the bus to arrive. Rush back into the house to retrieve forgotten homework pages. Kiss them goodbye and wave as the bus pulls away.

If I'm lucky, I can gulp down some coffee while I get dressed and before Mom wakes up and her daily care begins. Get her up and into a chair while I strip the wet sheets and blankets off her bed. Put clean bedding on. Wash her as best I can while she sits in the chair resisting the whole time. Thank goodness the home health aide will be here tomorrow. Hopefully she can get Mom into the shower for a thorough washing. Help her eat breakfast and take her morning meds. Once she's settled, launder the soiled linens before they begin to stink up the whole house.

I search the refrigerator and cupboards for something quick and easy to make for dinner. Spaghetti with sauce from a jar it is. Everyone is tired of it, but too bad. I'll add some garlic and mushrooms to help change it up, if I get the time.

Before I know it, it's time for Mom's lunch and a breathing treatment. Crap, she's wet again. A chair bath, clean sheets and clean gown. More laundry and another cup of coffee to keep me going.

Two hours later, the bus is here and I'm out of breath. The

43

phone rings. It's John, he has a dinner meeting tonight and will be home late. Kiss the kids goodnight for him. I go into the bathroom, turn the water on, and begin to cry.

Just for Today

Some days I feel like throwing in the towel. But then, I'd just have to pick it up again. – *Maxine*

Caregivers, just for today leave the towel where it landed. I know you are doing everything you can to maintain your home, your family, and the person in your care. You do much more for others than you do for yourself. Just for today let go of every little thing that doesn't have to be done right now.

Maybe you were taught to make your bed every day?

- Just for today, leave your bed unmade.
- Instead of cooking dinner, order a pizza.
- Let the dust settle on the coffee table. It will be there tomorrow.
- Stay in your pajamas.
- Let someone else take out the trash.

Consider the things you do automatically because you have always done them ... pick *at least* one ... and just for today let it go. Use those few moments to have a cup of coffee with Maxine and absorb a bit of her attitude. Do it just for today. Do it for you.

MIKE

I could not believe what was happening. I walked into the nursing home and there was Dad talking to one of the male aides. Not only talking, but smiling and moving his arms to punctuate whatever he was saying. What miracle was this? Or was I looking at someone who resembled my father. No, it was him. There was no doubt about it when he motioned me over and introduced me to his friend, Antonio.

"My son plays the drums," Dad said with pride. "All the time when he was growing up he's come in from school and start playing music. Not like in the Old County. Not good music like Anrdrea Bocelli or Caruso or Pavarotti. No, he plays today music. Some good, some sound like big noise, but he play it anyway. I like music. When I was in Italy we dance on Saturday night. The girls come, the boys come. We dance the waltz, tango, foxtrot. Music is good."

I agree music is good. I can't imagine life without music, but I still couldn't figure out what was going on with Dad. For weeks he hadn't spoken to anyone. He barely moved on his own, and now he was talking and remembered doing the tango over sixty years ago.

"It's the music," Antonio said. "It stays with us all through life, stored deep in the brain. We're just beginning to understand how it can help enhance the life of someone with dementia."

"This is awesome, music that I love is the language that will help me connect with my father and his memories. It's a miracle. Hey Dad, when you were dancing the tango with the pretty girls did you ever steal a kiss?"

45

"Not polite to kiss and tell," he said. But, by the twinkle in his eye I knew the answer was yes, and he was remembering it fondly.

The Sound of Music and Dementia

Sitting in the park on a recent summer night, listening to a local band playing music I danced to as a teen, I started to sing along. Singing isn't something I normally do, unless I'm alone in the car with the windows rolled up. I firmly believe it's best for everyone and if you ever heard me sing you would surely agree.

I felt safe singing in the open air, joining others like me overcome with the joy and nostalgia of our shared musical history. Before long, the band ramped things up and went into a medley of rock songs. Soon people were on their feet dancing. A little one, barely able to walk, moved to the beat, her tiny legs bouncing as she clapped with glee. Standing beside her, her grandparent's did the same.

"More!" She said when the music stopped. Her grandparents agreed.

The song that was playing that night may have become imprinted on her memory, just as it had on mine years before. Many years from now she may hear it and feel the same freedom she did that night. I hope so.

>❀<

Music speaks to us at every age and the music of our youth carries us back in time like nothing else can. I once told my husband that when my generation gets old instead of the songs of the forties and fifties heard in nursing homes now, the place will be rocking to the music of the Beatle's and the Rolling Stones. Women and men will smile as they remember holding their sweetheart and dancing to love tunes like My Special Angel by the Vogues or My Girl by the Temptations.

I didn't realize when I said it how true it would turn out to be. The music of the past can enhance the lives of the elderly, especially those with Alzheimer's and other forms of dementia and patients with Parkinson's disease.

My father-in-law was extremely introverted due to his long history of mental illness. When Parkinson's disease and dementia entered the picture things got worse. He often went days without speaking, and could become quite suspicious and hostile. One thing that always brought him out of his shell, at least for a while, was listening to opera. A special favorite of his was Andrea Bocelli. As soon as he would hear Bocelli begin to sing, his posture would change. Normally quite rigid in expression and movement he would begin to relax. First his shoulders would move away from his ears and his fingers, so often curled, would rest open on his knees. Then the smile would come, and he'd begin to speak of life in Italy and the days spent with his family there. He was a lighter, happier version of himself. The effects of the music usually lasted long after he indicated he'd heard enough. It was as if he became a bit of the man he once was. And each time it happened, it was a gift for him and for us.

KEVIN

I cried in the doctor's office this morning. I never cry. It's not manly. And what do I have to cry about? I have a good job, a great wife, and a nice home. My kids are all doing well. In a few years I'll be able to retire and do some traveling. Life is good. So what's the problem?

I don't know how to help my mom or my wife. I see them both fading. One sick and needing almost constant care, and the other wearing herself out be on call for Mom's needs day and night. I wish I could do more, but I can't be in two places at once. I need to go to work to pay the bills. I have to run the household errands on the weekends. I do what I can to help my wife in the evenings, but it's so little when the need is so great.

The guilt is overwhelming. When I'm at work my mind is on what's happening at home. When I'm home, I'm distracted by how much I didn't get done at work. I can hardly sleep for worrying and neither can my wife. We are snapping at one another all the time. We never did that before. It's not like us at all. Each time I hurt her feelings the guilt pours over me.

I took the day off today. My turn to take Mom to the doctor and give my wife some time to rest for a bit. The doctor said I looked worse than my mom and asked how I was doing. I told her I was fine. I didn't realize I was crying until Mom took a tissue out of the box on the doctor's desk and wiped my face with it.

How pathetic is that? I was supposed to be taking care of her, and she ended up taking care of me.

Dealing with the Guilt

I am, as usual, multi-tasking. I have one load of dirty clothes in the washing machine and one load of clean clothes running track in the dryer. I have the timer set to notify me when the pot of potatoes I set to boil will be done enough to mash for Dad's lunch, and I'm trying to remember where I put my cell phone. I don't want to have to scurry around looking for it when the nurse calls to discuss the continuing fluctuations in Dad's blood pressure.

And I'm trying to figure out how to deal with the guilt.

I wish I could be more like my friend, Dana. Dana does not multi-task. She claims that it takes less effort to do ten things consecutively than it does to try to do five things all at once, and she insists that feeling guilty is a complete waste of her time and energy.

"Get over it," she insists. "Guilt is a useless emotion."

Dana is probably right. I just don't know how she does it.

I can try to do fewer tasks at once, but I know I'll never get down to doing only one thing at a time. Not as long as Dad is alive. No matter where I am, or what I'm doing, part of my mind and most of my heart is with him. I go to sleep puzzling over how I can add flavor to his diet of pureed food and thickened liquids. I wake up wondering what his blood pressure reading will be. Sometimes I stop in mid step, listening to the too-still air, hoping for a small cough or sneeze to signal he's still breathing.

Caring for him reminds me of caring for my babies in the first days of their lives. A time when they seemed too fragile to be of this world, and I feared that any

49

misstep on my part would bring on disaster.

He had that heart attack last month. He almost died. Again. And I feel so guilty about that. Shouldn't I have seen the signs before it got that far? Looking back, he did seem more tired than usual, and his heart rate was slow enough for an alarm to be sent to his doctor through the tele-health monitor in our home. Still, everyone agreed he seemed to be doing fine. The readings weren't dangerously low.

"We know you're taking good care of him," his care coordinator said. "We'll keep an eye on this for a day or two and see what happens."

Now we know. A heart attack happened. I realize that his EKGs had been fine up to that day. I know he never complained of chest pain or shortness of breath until the moment the blood clot hit him. I know that I did the right thing when I called 911 right away.

"Time is critical in a situation like this," the paramedic explained. "And you got us here fast. You did good."

I don't feel good... I feel guilty. And I sit here today wondering how to deal with that. And I'm not the only one who feels it. Not by a long shot. My husband feels guilty because I spend most of my time caring for the man we both call Dad, his father. On an especially hard day, he will apologize many times. "My poor honey," he says. "I feel so guilty."

I keep telling him there is no reason for him to feel any guilt. He goes to work every day to earn the money that supports us so I can be at home with Dad. We planned for this long before it became necessary. We agreed on the division of labor. But still he feels it, and it shows in his face even when he doesn't say it out loud.

I understand. My own father, older than Mike's Dad

and also quite ill, is being taken care of by his stepson in Florida while I'm here taking care of someone not of my blood. I long to go to him, but I can't and he doesn't want to come here. Still I cringe every time I hear him say, "I don't know what I'd do without Brian." In my heart I feel that he's mine, not Brian's, and I should be with him. Shouldn't I?

A cousin of mine, so close we are more like sisters than actual cousins, feels guilty because her mother is being cared for by her daughter. Grandmother and granddaughter live in the same town and share a special bond. My cousin lives across the country, visits often and calls almost daily.

"She's doing what I should be doing. I feel such guilt," my cousin says even as she acknowledges that her life is in Florida and her mother will never leave New York where she was born and has lived all of her 82 years. I try to reassure her that things are just as they should be.

"There is nothing wrong with your daughter being there for your mother. It's what they both want, and she is in good hands. It's okay," I insist. But in my heart I feel guilty for not having a better answer for her.

Mike's dad, my father, and my aunt are all getting good care. The problem is not with them, it's with us. The caregivers. The ones who try to do it all and can't.

The timer on the stove has gone off almost simultaneously with the buzzer on the dryer. The phone is ringing and Dad is making his way down the stairs. I can deal with all that. That part's easy. But tell me, if you can. How do I deal with the guilt? How do I get over it?

I need to talk to Dana.

51

KAREN

I hate this disease. It's stolen my mother from me. I don't know who the hell that angry, foul mouthed bitch is, but she's not the woman who raised me.

She called me a fat whore this morning and that's the nicest thing she's said to me in days. I hate to admit it, but in that moment, I hated her, too.

I keep reading that it's the disease talking, not her. How do I know that? Maybe the loving, supportive, funny woman she used to be was all an act. What if what I'm seeing now is the real her. The one she kept hidden all these years. Her filter is gone and all the ugliness inside is coming out.

She's so angry all the time it's affecting me, triggering my own anger. I try to push it away, but it comes roaring back when she lashes out at me. Then, just when I feel as if I can't take it another minute, she smiles at me and I see her again as she used to be. Yesterday, she took my hand and said, "I love you, sweet girl."

"I love you, too, Mom," I said and we had a good afternoon together. She had forgotten what she'd said and done earlier. I had not.

It was the disease talking. The heat of my anger is almost gone, but traces remain. I wish I could believe it will not come back. I can't. What I do know is that I will always love her, no matter how mad I get.

Being Mad Doesn't Mean I Stop Caring

When I felt angry and resentful for the first time as a caregiver, it was devastating. Where was it coming from? Why was it coursing through me when the crises had passed and things were getting better?

What's wrong with me? I cried, and I prayed.

The guilt that accompanied those feelings threatened to overwhelm me. I didn't know if I could go on. If I should go on. I was ashamed of myself for being so weak.

What I didn't understand was that my feelings were normal. The anger was a passing storm sweeping away debris that had been piling up inside me. It was a way to release the stress and worry that comes with being a caregiver.

There is plenty to be mad about. These diseases affect the entire family. You get mad precisely because you care. So, yes, go ahead and get mad. Slam doors, stomp your feet, cry, curse if you want to. You've earned it.

BARBARA

I need sleep. It is not just rest I need. I need deep dreamless sleep. A quiet mind that renews the sprit and calms the soul. I never thought of it this way until now, but sleep is deeply spiritual. "Be still and know I am God," the Psalm says. To me sleep would feel very much like prayer. It is in the depths of our nightly rest that we are restored and in many ways, inspired, to carry on. When we are awake, the "what ifs," keep coming. Thoughts hop hither and yon, stumbling over one another, keeping us from seeing the solution that is magically revealed in the morning. I need that insight now more than ever.

I need sleep.

A Caregiver's Dream

One of the most common bits of advice for caregivers is to get a good night's sleep.

Goodnight. That simple word brings to mind a series of wonderful images. I close my eyes and see myself drifting off to sleep in the biggest most comfortable bed on the market. I'm covered with a whisper soft blanket. I'm hugging my pillow. A tiny smile hints at sweet dreams to come. When morning arrives, I will awake refreshed ready to face another day caring for my loved one.

That is what I am supposed to do, right? That's what all the experts said. Trust me, it's what I would have loved to do.

Enter reality:

"Goodnight, Dad."

"Goodnight."

It was eight o'clock in the evening and he had just had his last breathing treatment of the day. Only one round of medications was left to be taken. I had two hours to spend, alone with my husband. Exhausted, we were only half listening to each other. I kept one ear open in case Dad needed me. Nodding at my husband to indicate I was paying attention, I was also fighting to keep my eyes open.

At 10:00 PM I got up and took Dad his last medication of the night. He took it without complaint. Yea!

"Goodnight, Dad."

"Goodnight."

I was too tired to brush my teeth. Tomorrow was another day and I hadn't had much to eat anyway. Did I take a shower this morning? I couldn't remember. After saying my prayers, I closed my eyes and waited for sleep to come. My thoughts looped and circled around on themselves. *What ifs* and *why didn't I* competed with *I should have* until I finally lost consciousness.

12:15 AM – His bed alarm went off. He hated the alarm. He hated the bedside commode and he resented me for making him use them. I ran down the hall to discover he had scooted down to the foot of the bed and managed to squeeze through the space between the bedrail and the foot of the bed. He was clinging to the rail, trying to keep from falling.

"Here, let me help you." I eased him over to the commode and helped him stand to pee. He refused to sit. "I'm not a girl!"

"Why didn't you call me if you wanted to get up?"

"I didn't want to bother you. I used my short cut."

55

"Short cut?"

It took me a few moments to understand he was talking about the gap between the bedrail and the end of the bed.

"You aren't supposed to get up unless someone is with you. You could fall. That's why the doctor ordered an alarm for your bed."

"The doctor sent it?"

"Yes."

"I don't remember. How does he know if I go to the bathroom? It's none of his business."

Five minutes later we were both back in bed.

12:45 AM – His bed alarm went off. That time he tried to climb over the rail and was stuck half way over.

"What are you doing?"

"I have to pee."

I got him up and helped him to the commode. He stood for a couple of minutes. Nothing happened.

"I thought I had to go." We went back to bed.

2:00 AM – The bed alarm went off. He was stuck half way out of the bed again. We repeated the scene above.

2:10 AM – Alarm went off again. His foot is stuck in the rail.

3:05 AM – Alarm went off again. He had scooted down to the foot of the bed and was trying to get up.

"I have to pee." That time he did.

3:15 AM – Alarm went off again. "I'm thirsty." I went to the kitchen and mixed some thickener in water and helped him spoon it into his mouth.

4:00 AM – He was calling for me. I rushed to his room. His covers were tangled around him and he couldn't move. I got him into a chair and arranged his bedding. Had him pee while we were up.

5:15 AM – The bed alarm went off again. I knew I

was up for the day.

The next day, and the next, and the days after that? Repeat the above actions from the beginning. Sometimes it was the voices that woke him. Some nights he thought it was day and he was ready to start his routine.

Believe me, I followed all the suggestions. I kept him up during the day. It didn't matter. I put him in adult pull-ups so he didn't have to use the bedside commode. I'd find them torn to shreds the next time I went to his room. I followed all the advice about soothing music and quiet time before bed. I tried it all again and there we were night after night. Sometimes I made a bed for myself on the floor beside him so he knew he was not alone. Still the alarm went off through the night.

Get a good night's sleep? I was ready. I even drifted off for a while, and then his bed alarm went off. Again.

TONI

The first Christmas commercials are popping up on television. It's not even Thanksgiving yet. Halloween has barely passed. What a night that was. I didn't bother buying any treats and kept the porch light out to keep the little ghosts and goblins from ringing the doorbell. It broke my heart to do it, but with Hal sun-downing like he does I had no choice.

Every evening, when the sun begins to set, Hal gets agitated and begins to pace in his room. It doesn't matter how calm he's been during the day or even if he's dozed off in his chair watching television. It's uncanny how his mood changes. He mutters angrily to some unseen person, and if I approach he gets even more agitated. I've learned to close the blinds and curtains in his room before sunset. Sometimes it helps, often it makes no difference. Halloween is one of the nights when nothing helps. We simply ride it out as best we can.

At least he didn't end up in the hospital that night. There is something about the days I used to look forward to that sets him off. Christmas and Thanksgiving are the hardest. Every year at holiday time Hal gets sick, usually ending up in the hospital for several days. Why? I can't figure out. It's not as if he goes shopping and gets exposed to people coughing and sneezing all over him. He only leaves the house to see his doctors. I do my shopping online because I can't leave him alone.

Every year it's something, and somehow it sneaks up on me. I begin to relax thinking he's going to be fine this year, and at the worst possible moment, I learn just how wrong I am.

"Toni, I don't feel so good," he says, and off we go. Maybe next year will be different.

The Holidays Are Here - It's Time to Go to the Hospital

It happened every year. At some point in the holiday season, Rodger would be in the hospital. Aspiration pneumonia three years in row between Thanksgiving and Christmas. One year a heart attack on Thanksgiving Day. Worsening dysphagia on top of fluid buildup in his lungs due to congestive heart failure the following year. One time a broken partial plate sliced a gash in his tongue requiring a trip to the nearest Urgent Care. He sat with a bloody paper towel hanging out of his mouth for over an hour waiting for treatment while others in the waiting room tried hard not to stare. I can only wonder what they must have been thinking. A week later, he developed a fever and had to be admitted with an infection of unknown origin.

The stress of the Holidays got to him. We were doing all the work to get everything done while his routine went on unchanged. Why then did it take such a toll on him?

Holidays are a time to gather and share a feast with our family and friends. When we are children, we watch our mothers and grandmothers prepare the meal, inhale the delicious aromas of various pies baking in the oven, and look forward to chasing our siblings and cousins through the house while the adults sit at the table long after dinner and talk about boring stuff.

When we become the parents, we follow in their footsteps taking satisfaction in passing on our traditions. Then the losses begin, becoming more

59

devastating as the years pass. Our grandparents first, then our parents. We still celebrate, but the occasions are tinged with melancholy as we look back with joy and a few tears remembering the ones no longer with us. We share stories of the past. We laugh, and cry, and hold the new generation of infants and children a bit longer than they like because they are our hope. And we know one day, we will be their memories.

The stress of the Holidays got to Rodger every year. I wonder if it was because he was reliving the losses more than the joys of the season.

GRACE

She wants to go home. No, she demands to go home. How many times do I have to tell her this is her home? She's been here four years. She's the one who wanted to sell their house after Dad died. She planned to move in with me and put the money from the sale in her savings to pay for her care as she got older. It made sense. As an only child, all we have is each other.

It worked out great until she fell and broke her hip. The hip healed fine, but she was never the same after the operation. When she woke up she didn't know where she was or what had happened to her. She didn't recognize me for the first three days, and kept asking why her mother didn't come and get her.

The surgeon said anesthesia sometimes has this kind of effect on the elderly. No one told me that before this happened, but even if they had it wouldn't have changed the situation. She needed the surgery.

Some days are better than others. When she has a few good days in a row, I begin to hope that we are through the worst of it and she will be okay again. It never lasts though. Each time she comes back, she's lost more of who she used to be. Maybe that's why she wants to go home. She wants to return to a time and place where her mind is clear and the world makes sense. I don't blame her. If it were possible I'd help her pack her bags and go there with her.

I Want to Go Home

"Dad, you are home. Let me take you back to your room."

"No! I want to go home now! Let me out of here."

Caregivers hear these words and know they are in for a very difficult day or a long sleepless night. It doesn't matter how long Mom or Dad have been with them or even how long a husband or wife have lived in the same place. There often comes a time when a person with dementia insists they want to go home.

I understand the feeling. I don't have Alzheimer's or dementia but there were plenty of moments during the years I spent caring for Rodger that I longed to have someone take care of me again. More than once I softly whispered a little unrealistic prayer, "I want my mother."

I knew where I was. I knew there was no going back to the day when Mom had supper on the table and the biggest worry I had was how to get all my homework done or what grade I would get on the math test. And, truth be told, I didn't really want to turn back time. What I wanted, what I longed for in the moment, was to feel safe in a world that had become confusing and very different from what I wanted it to be.

Once I got where he was coming from, I told Rodger I'd like to go there someday and asked him to tell me all about it. Sometimes it worked, and he would settle down and talk about days gone by and holidays on the farm in Italy. I loved hearing the stories of his childhood and his mother's cooking. Sometimes it didn't work, and we both felt lost and alone. When that happened I would, again, find myself saying, "I want my mother."

JILL

I finally had a chance to see some of my friends yesterday. It's been months, and I was beginning to wonder if they remembered who I am anymore. No one calls or visits, not since I left work to take care of my sister. She had a massive stroke six months ago. Her right arm and leg are paralyzed and she has temporal lobe dementia. I looked it up online. I didn't know anything about vascular dementia and how different parts of the brain work. Boy, am I learning now.

Damage to the temporal lobe can affect personality, behavior, and language. That's what I found online. Her doctor confirmed it. Living with her confirms it every day. She didn't have any savings and her health insurance doesn't include long-term care. I quit my corporate job and now I work from home as a freelance writer. With my income and her disability payments we get by, barely. If I go a week without an assignment, its beans and rice for dinner until the end of the month.

Some days are so hard I don't know how much more of this I can cope with. She has aphasia. When she tries to speak to me, her words come out all jumbled and she gets mad when I don't understand what she needs. Then she starts cursing me in her language. I know she's swearing by her expression and the unmistakable gestures she makes with her left hand.

She can write a few words, but the order is all mixed up. For example this is what she wrote yesterday, "Eat, eat, breakfast me." Later she shoved this into my pocket. "Head strings flying. Fix you." It took me a long time to figure out that she wanted me to comb her hair.

That's what my life is like now, so I was thrilled when I received a long-awaited check and was able to hire a retired nurse to come and stay with my sister for a couple of hours.

I was really looking forward to lunch in a restaurant and some normal conversation. What I wasn't looking forward to was a lot of unsolicited, impractical advice. I know they meant well. So do all the people who tell caregivers to take a break and to take care of themselves first. I wanted to cry by the time my friends got through telling me what they would do in my situation and how tired I looked and that I was actually harming my sister by not going to the spa now and then or getting a manicure. I had to get out of there before I told them to shut the hell up and ended up with no friends at all.

I know they meant well. I just wish they would come by and see what it's like to do this. Maybe then they would offer help instead of judgment.

Please Stop Telling Caregivers to Take a Break

Almost every website or blog for caregivers includes a number of posts advising readers to take care of themselves. Most lists will include some version of the following:

- Get plenty of rest.
- Eat healthy.
- See your doctor regularly.
- Don't try to do it all yourself.

Some lists suggest a bit of pampering:

- Take a bubble bath.
- Get a manicure.
- Put on some music and dance your stress away.

- Put your feet up.
- Go on vacation

All of the above are excellent suggestions. When I was an in-home caregiver, I longed to follow their advice, and I believe the caregivers reading their posts did as well. I, also, know how hard it is to have well-meaning people tell you what to do. What caregivers wonder is why people expect them to add more to their already nearly impossible list of things to do.

I remember how exhausted I was as a new mom. I walked around the house in a sleep deprived daze, my hair uncombed, teeth unbrushed until late in the day. My clothes were often wrinkled and spotted with unidentifiable bits of stuff. I felt like crying much of the time.

Things were much different for the precious darlings in my care. They slept for hours during the day. Their tummies were full and their tiny sleepers were soft, warm, and clean. I often stared at them as they dozed, thanking God for bringing them into my life. I, also, remember that just as I was about to lie down and take a nap or grab a bite to eat, a heart wrenching wail would ring through the house and all thought of caring for me disappeared. People commiserated. Friends shared their own stories of caring for a newborn, and some kind people brought casseroles so I didn't have to cook. No one suggested I get plenty of rest, take a bubble bath, give myself a manicure or go on vacation. If they had, I would have either laughed or cried, depending on the moment. Eventually things did get better. The baby slept through the night, and so did I. My infant became a toddler and while life remained hectic it became manageable.

Replace the word mom with caregiver and a loved one's name for the infant in the passage above and you get an accurate picture of life for a caregiver. The difference is, for a caregiver the cycle is reversed, toddlers become infants and infancy can last for years.

Sleepless nights, hour or longer feedings, frequent changes of bedding and adult diapers, and tantrums become daily occurrences lasting for years not months. When I was able to get someone to come in for respite care, Rodger punished me by acting out for days or weeks afterward. Often his temporary caregivers gave in and allowed him to feed himself. He'd aspirate and end up with a respiratory infection that landed him back in the hospital. His medication schedule would be disrupted, and his daily routine would spiral so out of whack that he'd be a nervous wreck. Everything that went wrong, and every new thing introduced, caused some sort of regression, either physical or mental. It became more and more difficult to determine which was worse—going without respite care or dealing with the aftermath.

I knew I had to take care of myself. I knew I needed to rest, take a hot bath, see my doctor for a checkup, and go on a vacation with my husband. I knew the people offering advice meant well. What they didn't understand was how much it would cost me to do as they said. Or how guilty it made me feel knowing I had failed to do even that right.

JODI

A friend of mine called the other day, which I really appreciated. It's so nice when one of my friends reminds me that they still think of me. Of course, the call was cut short because I had to tend to Mother. "You're such a saint to do this, Jodi. God bless you," my friend said. Although I was flattered, her words did not ring true.

I am no saint. It is not saintly to love my parents. It is not saintly to hide my tears when one of them lashes out at me. I am not perfect. I am not a hero. I am simply a woman doing the best I can to help them and me figure out this new reality. I wonder if people say these things about me because they don't know what it's like to do what I do, or if it's a way to indicate it's not something they feel they can do.

Not everyone can be a fulltime caregiver. Not everyone should be a fulltime caregiver. There a lot of reasons for both scenarios. Some people need such a high level of care it can't be done at home. Some family members are already stretched to the limit financially. Others have small children that need their time and attention. There is no wrong answer to the question about home care or placement in a nursing home or memory care facility.

Every family, every potential caregiver, must decide what is right in their situation. The rest of us must support that decision. The simple fact is that no matter what you decide to do now, the situation may change as time goes on.

While I may seem like a saint today, that perfect person you would hope would care for you someday. You didn't see me yesterday when I was at the end of my patience, hanging on by a thread, and praying for the ability to figure out what to do next.

I am not perfect. I am trying hard to manage the unmanageable, and hoping that tomorrow will be a better day for both of us.

I AM NOT PERFECT

If I am able to help you understand anything I hope it is this:

We are human. We become angry sometimes. We feel resentful when others go off on vacation or simply out to dinner and we can't. We get sick and tired of hearing the same question over and over. We need sleep, and get cranky when we don't get enough. Our heart breaks when the one we are trying so hard to help accuses us of mistreating them or stealing from them. Or worse yet, don't remember who we are.

Some days we want to give in, give up, and let go so badly we nearly fall apart. And then we feel terrible. We doubt ourselves and become convinced we are bad people.

We are not. We are the caregivers. We are not perfect. We are human. We give all we have. And then give some more.

I am not perfect and neither are you. No one is. You are a caregiver, and because of you the one in your care will have many more good days than he or she would have otherwise. That is all any of us can ask of ourselves.

JAN

I think I am more broken than my husband despite the dreadful brain damage he suffered in that motorcycle accident. He never thought it would happen to him. He was always safety conscious. He had the best equipment he could get. He never took foolish chances weaving in and out of traffic as some riders do.

"It's the knuckleheads that get in trouble," he would say whenever I warned him to be careful.

He always came home to me just as he promised, and I began to believe it would always be that way. When the call came on that beautiful autumn afternoon, I was not prepared to be summoned to the emergency room. Once there, I was not prepared to hear the words, "catastrophic brain damage."

He is alive, but our life as we knew it is over, and I can't stand the pain. At first I was angry with him. He should not have gotten on the bike that day. He could have chosen to do so many other things. He could have spent the day with me. The boys were at scout camp, and we had a rare opportunity to be alone for the weekend. Disappointed that he chose to go for a ride rather than go to see a film I'd be waiting to see, I hid my feelings and kissed him goodbye. After he left, I went to the store and picked up everything I needed to fix his favorite meal. I set the table with the good china and arranged the supermarket flowers that looked better than their price tag would suggest. Candles in the silver holders we received as a wedding gift added the final touch.

The call came before the steaks made it out of the package.

It was months before he was strong enough to leave the rehab center. I'm sure they are freezer burned and not worth thawing now. I think I would choke on mine anyway. I'll toss them in the trash in the morning.

I need my best friend to help me through this. Unfortunately, he is in no condition to offer his support. The drunk driver who sped through the red light took so much from him it takes all he has to get through the day. When that motorcycle skidded across the pavement breaking his bones and sending his brain bouncing around in his skull, it shattered my heart as well. I just hadn't realized it yet.

Tipped Over by Life

> When you find yourself tipped over by the gusts of life; when you fall to the floor and shatter, there are those who will walk around your pieces, lest they cut themselves upon the scatter. But others will pick up your broken bits, they'll cherish all they can gather. These are the ones to whom you must hold on forever, not the ones who forsook you, but the ones who glued you back together.
>
> —*Shakieb Orgunwall*

Caregivers, and those in their care, have been tipped over by the gusts of life. Many of our loved ones have fallen and broken bones. Many more have memories break away, piece by piece, creating razor sharp shards of anger and leaving resentment in their place. They lash out at us in their confusion and inadvertently cause us to begin to break as well.

Some fail to see the damage these devastating diseases bring about. Too often others see it and choose to "walk around the pieces, lest they cut themselves upon the scatter."

Caregivers, hold on to the ones who will be with you throughout this time, the ones who will glue you back together as often as you need it.

LIZ

That's it, I'm done. It's too hard. He's entitled to respite care. It's one of his benefits as a 100% disabled veteran. We were promised we could admit him to the hospital for up to thirty days each year but no more than fourteen days in a row.

I'm not asking for thirty days. I don't want fourteen days. There is no way I want him in there that long. It's bad enough when he has to be admitted for more than a day or two. He says it doesn't bother him, they like him there. I'm sure they do. He does everything he can to hide his symptoms, and tells the medical personnel to go take care of the sick people. He can take care of himself. Ha! He can take care of himself all right. He hides his medication in his cheek and spits it out when they aren't looking. He convinces them he needs Milk of Magnesia for nonexistent constipation throwing his entire system off. When he does get home, he punishes me for days by acting out and threatening to call and report me for holding him hostage. I do everything I can to keep him out of the hospital. But it's been months since I've had a break and I can't go on like this.

I need a weekend or two days and nights to rest and get some of my strength back. I had another panic attack last night. At least I know what they are now. The first one scared the wits out of me. I thought I was having a heart attack. Once the paramedics determined it wasn't that and my heart was fine, one of them asked what was going on that had me so stressed. When I told her I was a caregiver she understood. I didn't tell her about the migraine headaches that sent spikes of pain through my head more and more often, or about my hair that falls out in the shower these days. If it keeps up I'm going to be bald while he still has a head full of hair.

I kept calling and telling his case manager I needed to bring him in. He or she, depending on the day, kept telling me there were no beds available. Not knowing what else to do, I prayed. "Show me the path you want me to take."

The next morning, when I was given the same runaround, I lost it and told them to find a room or I was calling my congressperson and reporting the VA hospital was denying a benefit to a disabled veteran. Two hours later, I received a call saying a bed would be available in two days, and he could stay as long as I needed him to.

Sometimes God works in mysterious ways, and for that I am grateful.

I Can't Do This Anymore

I felt that way so many times in the seven years I spent as a caregiver for Rodger. I cried and vented and wished for more wisdom daily. I saw every setback, every new symptom, and every dreadful new diagnosis as a sign of failure on my part.

Scalded by guilt, worn down by his refusal to trust me, I resented him. Fearing where this spiral would take us and knowing any chance of respite care was weeks away, I began to pray. There were no miracles for us. He was not cured. I did not develop the patience of a saint. But it helped me understand again that he and I were not alone. And in that moment that's exactly what I needed.

Dear God,
Enlighten what is dark in me,
Strengthen what is weak in me,
Mend what is broken in me,

Bobbi Carducci

Bind what is bruised in me,
Heal what is sick in me,
And lastly,
Revive whatever peace and love has died in me.
Amen

BOBBI

Are You Sure You Want to Do That?

When I first told people that my ill father-in-law was coming to live with us the most frequent comment was, "Are you sure you want to do that?"

People didn't hesitate to tell me how hard it was going to be or how concerned they were about what would happen to me if I took on such a demanding role.

They were correct. The seven years I spent as caregiver for Rodger were some of the most difficult in my life. It did take a toll on me. I spent hours praying and crying and second guessing myself, and his many illnesses progressed until the inevitable happened, and he passed away. Now I write about those experiences as a way to help others who are caring for loved ones at home.

One question I hear now is, "Would you do it again?" And my response is an unequivocal, "Yes." The reason I say that is the same one I gave to the people who first questioned my decision to bring him into our home.

"I'm setting an example for my children." I answer; watching them pause to consider their own circumstances down the road.

What I didn't know at the time was that Rodger would be setting an example for us.

Rodger was diagnosed as paranoid schizophrenic in his twenties. He died on his 83rd birthday. Like most schizophrenics he was very gentle and so introverted he was almost reclusive. Days went by when the only words he spoke are "Good morning," and "I'm going for a walk." But every now and then he'd say, "I'm a lucky man," and that was my cue to settle in and listen. It may have been the umpteenth time I heard a story or it may have been something surprising and new, it didn't matter. My purpose was to bear witness.

We live in a world where people are consumed by want and infatuated by the manufactured need for the latest clothing, hot car, or designer pet. For people like us, he was an inspiration.

"I always had food when I was hungry and a job when I needed one. I never thought I'd be able to raise a family," he whispered, tears shining in his dark eyes. "But I was lucky. I was finally able to do it." And he did it amazingly well on a modest laborer's salary.

"You need luck to survive in this world," he said.

He came to the United States at the age of nineteen. His degree from an Italian university would only take him so far even in this land of opportunity. He decided to enlist in the Army and go to college on the G.I. bill. He was a lucky man.

He fell ill while serving overseas. In the 1950's treatment for the mentally ill included shock treatments and straight jackets. Well intentioned experimental therapies often did more harm than good. Many men died, others remained hospitalized forever. He was one of the lucky ones. After thirteen years of advances in medical treatment he left the hospital, got a job, married and raised a family. Modern medicine saved him. Courage, dignity and grace sculpted him into an heroic figure.

Before dementia, Parkinson's disease, and a bad heart made it impossible, people were used to seeing see us during his daily walk through the neighborhood. He loved sitting on the bench in the front yard watching the birds. When he was able, he insisted on helping out around the house. He brought a special grace to our home. He was a lucky man; he knew what was really important in this world. He was setting an example for his children.

Would I do it again? You bet I would.

ANTHONY

I hate coming here. He doesn't know me anymore. Yet I am drawn here each week to ease my mind. I have to make sure he is being cared for. He would hate it here, too. If he knew where he was. It's weird seeing my brother in the same place our grandfather lived before he died.

"If I ever end up like that just take me out in the woods and shoot me," he said. I ignored it, but his wife could not.

"Don't say that. I don't want to live without you," she insisted.

She didn't have to. Breast cancer took her three years before he got sick. Sometimes when I enter his room he's talking to her. Although it breaks my heart, I can understand his wanting to relive their life together. They were happy. Who wouldn't prefer that to this place?

It's all the other days that make it almost unbearable. The days when he speaks only gibberish. The sounds run together in a rapid cadence while he slaps his forehead over and over. Where he is in those moments is nowhere I ever want to be. What are the voices saying? Who are they? What are they? I hope I never find out. I hate coming here.

Hearing Voices When No One is There

Many people hear voices when no-one is there. Some of them are called mad and are shut up in rooms where they stare at the walls all day.

78

Others are called writers and they do pretty much the same thing.

—*Margaret Chittenden*

Little did I know when I first read that quote how true it is or how the voices of mental illness and creativity would come together in my life.

Rodger heard the voices of mental illness. Diagnosed with paranoid schizophrenia as a young man they often spoke to him. I hear the voices of my characters. As I write our story I rely on his voices and mine to bring it to life.

I knew he was a bit odd long before he came to live with us. His life centered on meals and his three daily walks. His social life was almost nonexistent. He attended weddings and funerals if pressed to do so by his wife, and he barely tolerated visits from family. Other than that, he spent his days in front of the television watching news programs and reruns of old westerns. I liked him, but I didn't know him very well. Even years after becoming his daughter-in-law, we had nothing more than a very superficial conversation and then he turned inward again.

"Hi. How's everything. How are the kids? How is work? That's good."

He was the same with everyone no matter how closely related or how long it had been since he'd seen them.

Married for over forty years, my in-laws had a contentious relationship, yet it worked for them. I believed that once the worst of his grief over losing her eased, he would like living with us. Mike and I would provide a loving and safe home where he would finally be able to relax in peace and quiet. I didn't know the voices were already working against me.

❧ ✻ ☙

I was putting the last touches on dinner, and called his name to let him know it was almost time to eat when he ran out of the house and down the street in a panic.

"She's trying to kill me! I can't trust her!" he told the sheriff's deputy who happened to live nearby. Seconds later, I arrived beside them; out of breath from running after him while praying I'd be able to catch him before he had a heart attack.

That was the beginning of years of cat and mouse games where I tried to do everything I could to save him from himself. And he did everything he could to resist my efforts.

I tried to understand what was happening.

"What do the voices say?" I asked.

"They say what they say."

"How do you feel when they speak to you?"

"Nervous and suspicious."

"Suspicious of what?"

"Suspicious. That's it."

He refused to say more. Eventually I could tell when the voices were there.

"The others are active today," I would say to myself. Although he got his daily medication on time, crushed and mixed into applesauce, more and more often it wasn't enough to keep them quiet.

"Is this food any good?" he asked one day before lowering his head to sniff his plate. I thought he was concerned that something had spoiled after the power had been knocked out by a severe storm. I assured him it was fine.

"She's poisoning me slowly," he told the nurse on his next visit to the hospital. "It's not her fault. She has to do what the boss says."

"Who is the boss?" I asked.

"The boss is the boss. He controls everything. Don't let her kill me."

After taking antipsychotics for over sixty years, the medication was losing the ability to work.

"There may come a time when it doesn't work at all," his doctor warned. As much as I did not want to lose him, I prayed God would take him before that happened. He often said that when the time came he wanted to die at home. If there was a way we could make that possible, we would.

"Does he ever tell you what they say to him?"

"He won't talk about that."

"Based on his behavior when off his medication, in his case, they're not saying anything good. Often they are screaming at him when you're talking to him. If he doesn't respond to you, or refuses to believe what you tell him, it could be because he's been warned not to. It could also be that he doesn't understand what you're saying because he's hearing several voices at the same time," the doctor said.

I can relate to that last part. I tune everything out when a new character starts clamoring to have his or her story told. It's never frightening, but it can be very confusing when a multitude of ideas start coming more rapidly than I can sort them out. It may take my husband several tries to get my attention when this happens.

"Earth to Bobbi."

"Hmmm? Did you say something?"

"Okay, I get it. The others are here again."

Mike teased me about 'the others' but it's true. The voices of my characters are often as real to me as Rodger's voices were to him. And now Rodger's voice is the one I hear as I write our story. Sometimes what he says isn't very nice, reminding me of the difficult days we shared. And sometimes his message is a touching reminder of why our time together was such a gift.

"Welcome back," I whisper.

>�֍<

When Rodger was hearing voices, I was careful not to confront him. As long as he didn't act out in a way that could be dangerous to him, or others, I didn't interfere. If he became restless or combative I followed doctor's orders and gave him a prescribed sedative.

When I hear the voices in my head, I sit at my desk and let the story flow, just as I'm doing now. Perhaps that's what keeps me sane.

MARY

When I was a teenager, I would always cringe when Dad would tell one of his corny jokes to my friends, or worse yet, my dates. I don't know where he came up with most of them. Each one was worse than the one before. Whenever I begged him to stop, he'd say," Come on, Sugar Plum, that was funny and you know it."

Sometimes I did laugh, and that was all the proof he needed to find more material for his one man comedy routine.

"If I can make at least one person smile every day, I have done something to brighten the world."

It wasn't until I was an adult dealing with all the responsibilities and challenges that entails that I began to appreciate the gift he had, and how right he was. Whenever I needed a lift, I'd find a reason to call him. Just hearing his voice when he answered the phone saying, "Why hello there, Sugar Plum," lifted my spirits. But no matter how long we talked, we both knew the conversation wasn't over until he cleared his throat, and said, "Wait until you hear this one." What followed was either a new joke he's picked up somewhere in his daily travels or an old chestnut I'd heard a thousand times. The old ones eventually became our favorites, especially when I began to say the punch lines with him and we'd both laugh. Now he's in a nursing home and he may not remember where he is, but he still greets everyone he sees with a smile and a joke.

I love you, Dad.

Be the Reason Someone Smiles Today

Even if it's you. Even if you have to work at it. And even as hard as it is being a caregiver. As devastating as it could be in so many ways, there were moments when I couldn't stop the giggles. And laughter, like a good cry, can make it possible to go on. And sometimes the humor comes at the most unexpected times.

❧ ❀ ☙

When Dad first came to live with us, the only things he asked us to buy for him were Milk of Magnesia and prune juice. He had prescriptions for stool softeners and laxatives issued by his former doctors and continued by his new doctor. He constantly complained of constipation, greeting everyone he spoke to, including strangers, with, "Hello. How's everything? My bowels don't move." If he did happen to go, he made sure he told them about that as well, in great detail. It soon became clear he was taking far too much of the stuff. Every day, in the morning and at midday, he'd drink a large glass of prune juice, followed by Milk of Magnesia. Often he'd wait a few moments after taking it, look at his watch, and take some more. A few moments later he'd do it again. One day, after just telling me he'd had a bowel movement, I saw him drink another large glass of prune juice and then reach for the Milk of Magnesia.

"Why are you taking that? " I asked.

"For the constipation," he said.

"But you just went."

"That don't count. It was all liquid."

That's when I knew I had to do something. No matter how we tried to explain it to him, he wouldn't accept that the laxatives were causing his problem. The more he took, the worse it got—and the more he worried—resulting in a vicious cycle that was interfering in his normal bodily functions. His psychiatrist said that it's not unusual for a schizophrenic to keep track of what goes in and out of his body. In his mind, solid food was going in but nothing solid was coming out. That meant something was very wrong. Once I began to limit his access to prune juice and Milk of Magnesia, and started monitoring his use of laxatives, he started showing signs of stress. He paced and muttered to himself and began making frequent trips to the bathroom where he'd sit for hours, waiting for something to happen. I hated to see him like that, but I had to ease him off the stuff. His doctor tried to help by telling him that taking too many laxatives could interfere with his other medications and land him back in the hospital. He wasn't buying it. When I wouldn't give in, he complained to my husband, and when he backed me up, Dad called him one of the worst insults he could think of.

"You're nothing but a dictator! You're another Mussolini, that's what you are!"

Later, after he calmed down and we were getting ready for bed, my husband looked over at me and shook his head. "Mussolini? Now I'm Mussolini?"

I couldn't hold it in any longer. The giggles I'd been trying hard to stifle came rolling out. "The Mussolini of laxatives!" I laughed harder. "You Fascist poop dictator!"

He looked at me in confusion for a moment, and then the hilarity of the situation hit him and he was laughing as hard as I was. I laughed so hard I got the hiccups, and that made us laugh even more. We ended up rolling on the bed, laughter feeding more laughter, until we were exhausted.

"Oh, wow, I needed that," I said when I was finally able to catch my breath.

"Me too," he agreed. "I don't know how you do it every day. He's so damned stubborn. I'm glad I'm not like that."

"Right." I poked him the ribs. "Me either. I'm not stubborn. I'm determined."

"Yes, dear," he said with a grin. "Do you think you can determine to keep loving me through all this?"

"Sure, if you can determine to come over here and give me a kiss."

"You got it, Babe." And he did.

HANA

Most of the time my father-in-law is oblivious to what day it is. He used to make my mother-in-law furious every year when she had to remind him several times to buy her an anniversary card. It was also the one time each year that they went out for dinner and saw a movie together. He hated it. She insisted on it.

"What you need a card on birthday or anniversary for?" he would ask. "You born, so what? We all got born. We all gonna die someday. You know when we marry. I know when we marry. You don't need a card for that."

"Just go," she would insist. He would go.

I'll never forget the time I was visiting and he walked in and handed her a card. When she opened it she went rigid for a few seconds. Her face flushed such a deep shade of purple I thought she was having a heart attack.

'What the hell is this," she demanded.

"It's a card. You want a card, I get you one."

"Look at this! This is what he brings me on our anniversary." She thrust the card into my hands.

It was lovely. There was a beautiful flower arrangement on the front. At first, I didn't understand why she was upset. Then the words printed in a flowing script came into focus, and I knew then she wasn't in danger of dying, but he might be.

English was his second language, and while he spoke very well, reading and writing were difficult for him. I imagined him walking into the pharmacy and going to the card display looking for something suitable to make her happy. Seeing one with a large bouquet of white roses he may have thought, "Roses. She likes roses, I give her this one." She told him to get a card. She didn't say he had to read it.

I had to bite my lip and stifle my strong urge to laugh. She was not at all ready to see the humor in receiving a card on her wedding anniversary inscribed with the words, "With Our Deepest Condolences."

Happy Birthday

Today is my birthday. In a few hours my husband will be home and we'll share a special dinner. I'll open my present along with the last of the many birthday cards he's stashed around the house for me to find throughout the day.

My gift has been sitting on the dining table since the day before.

"Look," he whispered, pointing the way as if I'd get lost between there and the kitchen.

"Wow, what could it be?" I played along, knowing his delight in surprising me.

"Guess!"

"Is it a puppy?" I asked wide-eyed with fake anticipation. (Neither one of us would dream of bringing a puppy into our home at this time. We have our hands full already.)

"Nope, guess again."

It didn't take me long to convince him I was a terrible guesser and for the two of us to decide I'd just have to wait until today to find out what's in the pretty package wrapped in printed paper suitable for a baby shower.

"It was either that or Christmas paper," he grinned.

I like the baby shower paper. Our daughter is

expecting her first baby in November and it's nice to be reminded of the joy to come while celebrating my birthday. I stop to touch it each time I pass by on my way to put another load of laundry in the washer.

❧ ❀ ☙

It's been a busy morning. Dad started pacing at 6:00 AM. A dream, a memory or something on the news made him anxious.

I knew well before I strapped on the blood pressure cuff that the reading would be high. 190/100 was the first reading. After morning meds it dropped a bit to 180/90. A half hour later, his standing blood pressure held steady at 156/85. We'll settle for that. His heart is so damaged that we aim for acceptable, recognizing that optimum is no longer possible.

The bronchitis that plagued him for the last two weeks is finally gone. We both breathe easier now. While dusting his room, I discovered he'd removed the bulb from the lamp on his bedside table and placed it on top of a note he'd written.

"The bolb [sic] is still good. The ting that turns on is no good no more. Tell him." By him he meant his son, my husband, the one who, according to Dad, does everything around here."

I left a return message promising to let "him" know about the broken "ting" as soon as he gets home. I saw Dad in there a little while ago, reading the message, and nodding his head in approval. Note writing is something new. I don't know why he chose to tell me about the problem that way, but I'll be watching for more notes in the days to come.

❧ ❀ ☙

I had to take a bit of a break from writing when the florist delivered a beautiful bouquet of spring flowers. The colorful mix of variegated tulips, yellow roses, day

89

lilies and hydrangeas are accented by sprigs of a purple flower I can't identify. It's from my daughter and son-in-law. The card says, "Happy Birthday, Momma. I love you." I smile as I read the simple message that says so much.

"Happy Birthday to You," Dad sang out clearly when I showed him the flowers. Touched, I took his hand in mine and thanked him, tears coming to my eyes. I hadn't realized he was aware it was my birthday.

"The flowers are very beautiful. Enjoy them while you can," he said, removing his hand from mine. "You may be dead before your birthday comes again."

So much for our tender moment, I thought, and I watched him walk away. But he's right. Isn't he? We all need to enjoy each special moment as it comes, recognizing that the future may not be ours to see. So... Happy Birthday to Me. I'm off to smell the roses.

DIANE

I get it, he's sick. His brain is damaged by Alzheimer's disease, but I don't know how much of this I can take. My fastidious husband has turned into a belching, farting, stranger, who seems to delight in cutting loose whenever the urge hits him. And that's not all. His table manners are nearly nonexistent. If I don't watch him he won't bother to use a fork. He'll shovel food in with his hands and then wipe them on his shirt.

It was a relief when he said he didn't want to wait until seven o'clock to eat dinner anymore. He wants his meal at four, now. At least I don't have to hear him slurp and groan through the meal, and I can dine in peace.

I remember when sitting across the table from him was one of the best parts of my day. I long, not only, for the elaborate holiday meals we used to prepare together for our family and friends, but for one more simple meal with him the way it used to be.

Easter Dinner

My father-in-law is very down to earth. He doesn't need or desire finery or frills of any sort. He moves through the world with a childlike innocence.

"People's bodies make noises," he will tell you with no sense of unease at all. If a loud belch punctuates the end of a meal, he'll say, "If I don't let it out; I'll sussplode."

91

So there I was in the kitchen, where meals and memories are made in every home, and where many of us will gather in a few days to share Easter dinner with family and friends, thinking about the occasion.

In our house the meal consists of traditional baked ham, green bean casserole, mashed potatoes and gravy, *and* lasagna, in honor of the Italians in our midst. We'll add some Polish cookies that the Pittsburgh contingent insists on. They go surprisingly well with an assortment of Easter candy.

One year saw the introduction of a very strange concoction called Grandma's gravy. It came into the family along with our new son-in-law, and consists of pan drippings, canned gravy, orange juice and Lord knows what else. I may never develop a taste for it, but hey... somebody's Grandma made it, and that means it is welcome on my table.

What we're guaranteed during a meal like this is the lively sharing of cultures and memories. After dinner we will settle onto sofas and chairs in the family room, and before long, someone will burp loudly. No one will explode.

FRANK

Just once I'd like to hear him say, "Thank you." I know he's my dad, and I owe him respect, but I am his son—not his servant. "Get me a drink. Are you going to feed me today? Get in here, the TV don't work no more." That last one, after he's pushed every button on the remote control and it takes me several minutes to figure out how to fix the mess he's created.

He doesn't appreciate anything we do for him. No one else offered to take care of him. Some avoid him altogether, yet he acts like we owe him something for disrupting his life. He thinks we don't know how he watches from his room. We see him peeking through the open crack he leaves in his door. We hear him close it when we get near. I don't know what he thinks he's going to discover. All he's ever seen us do is watch a television show or do some household chore. He may have heard us complain about him once in while, but there is no getting around that. He's a handful, even on his good days.

I know this is even more difficult for Sue. My wife is a saint to put up with him all day. At least I get to escape to the office five days a week.

"Hey, get me a snack, I'm hungry, she don't make enough food."

Sue looks as if she's about to cry. A little over an hour ago, he chastised her for putting too much on his plate.

"How am I supposed to eat all this?" he demanded, before shoveling in every bite.

"I'll get him a snack," I tell my wife. "You've done enough for him today."

"Thank you. I'm beat. I can usually shrug it off when he says things like that, but tonight it's getting to me. Just once I'd like to hear him say, "Thank you.""

Easter With Rodger

The aroma of pasta sauce and roasting chicken wafted through the house. A beautiful apple pie rested on the kitchen counter. I hummed "Here Comes Peter Cotton Tail" as I adjusted my best tablecloth before going to the china cabinet and getting three place settings: dinner plate, salad plate, and bread plate. After carefully placing the proper utensils next to the plates, I added a water glass, and a delicate wine goblet, and then stepped back to admire the table. Mike had folded cloth napkins into delicate winged swans to place in the center of the dinner plates. Silver candlesticks flanked a beautiful flower arrangement that complimented the décor perfectly. Just before calling the men to dinner, I'd cut the pie, and placed three pieces on matching dessert plates, ready to be served when the time came.

Rodger had looked pleased when Mike and I went into his sitting room and presented him with his Easter basket that morning.

"Happy Easter," we greeted him.

"Happy Easter," he replied. "What's all this?"

"It's some Easter candy to sweeten your day," I said.

"They don't have Easter candy in the old country. Easter is a religious day. Everybody goes to church," Rodger said.

"It's a religious holiday for people here too," I explained. "But we also have the traditional Easter baskets."

"Do I have to go to church?" he asked. "I only go to

church when somebody marries or dies."

"You don't have to go to church if you don't want to," Mike assured him. "Enjoy your candy, and join us later for dinner in the dining room. Bobbi is making a special dinner."

"Who's coming? Do I have to take a shower?"

"No one is coming. It will be the three of us. But it would be nice if you took a shower. You'll be nice and clean for dinner."

"I don't need to take a shower to eat. I don't need special food. I eat anything."

"We know you'll eat anything," I said. "But on holidays we like to have a special meal. And you don't have to take a shower today, but you will have to take one soon. You need it. I'll call you when dinner's ready."

I could tell he was curious, something was going on. When he came down to go for a walk, he saw the table set in the dining room. He didn't say anything, but spent several minutes looking at it before he went out.

Even the weather was cooperating. The air was warm and the sun was shining. After his walk, Rodger sat on his bench in the front yard, watching the birds flit between the two feeders hanging from the tree he'd watched grow from the day we moved in.

He had become a fixture in the neighborhood by taking his three daily walks. He knew when people were moving in, and when a house was listed for sale. He kept track of who had dogs, and if they barked when he passed by, or not. He always let me know when anyone planted something new in their yard, and when the Christmas decorations went up. He rarely spoke to anyone, but he knew who lived where, and could tell if they'd changed their routine in any way.

Despite his earlier protest, when I called the men to dinner, Rodger arrived freshly showered and shaved, wearing clean clothes and a shy smile.

"Sit here, Dad," Mike said as he pulled out the chair at the head of the table.

"Me, here?" he asked.

"Yes, you're the guest of honor today."

"Guest of honor. I'm not a guest of honor. I'm not special."

"You are to us," Mike and I said at the same time.

Rodger didn't speak as he filled his dish with chicken and pasta. Nor did he say anything when I passed him a plate of salad, and offered him some toasted garlic bread from the napkin-covered serving dish.

"Before we eat, let's have a toast. Your wine glass has sparkling grape juice so you can drink too," Mike told his father. "Happy Easter," he said, raising his glass. "And to Rodger," he added.

I lifted my glass to my father-in-law, and repeated Mike's toast.

"To Rodger. We're so pleased you joined us to celebrate today. You look very nice."

"Thank you," he said. Then he lifted his fork and began to eat.

Everyone was quiet for several minutes, each lost in thought, and enjoying the meal. Rodger broke the silence, and Mike and I were stunned to see tears in his eyes.

"I never thought I'd have a meal like this, in a place like this. Everything so beautiful. The food, the dishes, flowers and candles. Everything. I feel like a big shot."

Dabbing at his eyes with his napkin, he looked around the room, and pointed at the delicately carved chairs and the gleaming china cabinets. He took a few moments to gaze at the framed print hanging on the wall. The print, *Dinner at the Ritz,* shows a group of

Victorian ladies dining, in their finery, at flower-laden tables on a summer afternoon.

"Beautiful ladies," he said. "Everything so nice. I never thought I'd have anything like this. I can't believe I'm going to die here. I was born in a big house, and I'm going to die in a big house. Thank you."

TINA

All I can think about when I see my mom like this is Dustin Hoffman in the film, *Rain Man*. Everything by the clock, no exceptions. Breakfast at seven, snack at ten-thirty, lunch at precisely twelve noon. Another snack at two. Her supper must be in front of her at six. Even five minutes late brings on a meltdown. The same is true of the rest of her day. Her favorite programs on television must not be preempted or delayed by a special report, no matter what disaster may be looming. She would probably bitch for days if a tornado interrupting a Dr. Phil rerun, and do it from her cot in the emergency shelter after the house had been reduced to rubble.

She even monitors my day. Monday is the day the laundry is washed, dried, ironed if needed, and put away. She will let me know if a single wrinkle is left on any item of her clothing.

Tuesday the first floor is dusted. Wednesday the second floor gets the same treatment. Thursday and Friday are for vacuuming each floor. Saturday the bathrooms are cleaned. Sunday is a day of rest. She doesn't realize it's also the day I precook most of her meals in order to guarantee her demanding schedule is met.

She monitors when I get the mail, and demands to see what is in every package delivered to the house. Then she scolds me for spending too much money. It doesn't matter that most of the boxes are refills of her various prescriptions and other items needed for her care, like Depends and compression hose.

The only time her routine, and now mine, can vary are the days I take her to the doctor. How pathetic am I? I now look forward to these visits. It's more work for me, getting her ready to go, and into the car with her walker, but it's a few hours out of the house. And if I'm lucky, a few moments in the sun and fresh air when we make our way from the car to the office. Once done, I get her back in the car and head for home, hoping to make it time for another rerun of Dr. Phil—or face the consequences.

I wonder how she keeps track of all these things when the rest of her short term memory is gone. Can anyone tell me that?

It Don't Make Sense

He was pacing. I could hear the floor squeak each time he reached the spot just outside his bathroom door. Three more steps and then he'd turn and go back the other way. Pace, pace, pace, squeak. Pace, pace, pace, squeak. Over and over.

Eventually he'd come down the stairs, and peer out every accessible window, checking to see if the rain had stopped and he could go out for a walk. I had to be on guard until it did. His need to follow his daily routine was so strong that if the rain didn't stop soon, he'd convince himself it wasn't that bad, and head out anyway. Despite all the reports that people don't get sick from getting chilled and wet, I worried that he'd get pneumonia. He couldn't afford another bout. It nearly killed him the last time. We were in for a long day.

I tried not to complain. I knew I had it easier than many caregivers. At that time, he could still walk and talk. He dressed and fed himself. And, although he needed to be reminded often, he was able to take a shower on his own with the aid of a shower seat, safety handles, and the handheld shower head. I was grateful for those things even as I prepared for the day when all that would change.

At eighty-one he was frail, and his list of aliments was long. The major ones were Parkinson's disease, emphysema, heart trouble, hypertension, short term memory loss, the onset of dementia, and the paranoid schizophrenia that had defined his life since his diagnosis at the age of twenty-three. The more minor ones, (the ones he liked to pretend didn't exist) included: swallowing problems, chronic toenail infections, diminished hearing and poor eyesight. And just to spice things up, we had what I called, "stubborn, old Italian disease" to deal with. It's a mix of ailments which required a team of doctors, a busy schedule of office visits, and strict monitoring of his medication.

"It's still raining," he said, "It don't make sense. It rained yesterday."

I didn't tell him that yesterday it was bright and sunny. If it had rained "yesterday" in his mind, that was his reality, and I went with it. If I didn't, his agitation would grow until it reached the point where he'd reject everything I said, and become convinced I was trying to trick him. From there it was a short hop to full blown paranoia, and the need for a sedative. The drug left him so listless, and out of it, I tried to avoid using it as much as possible.

"Well, the flowers and the grass need rain. Rain is good sometimes, isn't it?" I asked.

"Yes, rain is good for the flowers...good for the grass...I can't go for a walk. It don't make sense. It rained yesterday," he whispered softly. He turned and headed for the door.

"Dad, it's not time for your walk yet," I called to him, easing my body between his and the door. "You took a walk after breakfast, remember? We can go out this afternoon when sun comes out."

He paused for a moment, his head tilted as he tried

100

to decipher what I said.

"Yeah, I took a walk after breakfast. I remember now." He smiled and nodded at me before slowly walking toward his room."

It didn't matter that the walk he took after breakfast occurred yesterday. At that moment, he remembered the warmth of the sun on his face, and the pleasure of following a familiar routine. He was content, and his world made sense. And for a while... until he came back down and tried again...that was enough for both of us.

PAUL

I wish I'd never agreed to do this. I don't want to hate my father, but sometimes the anger I feel comes so close to hate it scalds me inside. He lies about taking his medicine. I came in from the store the other day and saw him looking out of the window over the kitchen sink, his pill box open on the counter. As I watched, he emptied the pills into his hand and put them in his pocket. Hearing me enter, he took a sip of water and turned toward me.

"What are you doing?" I asked.

"Time for my pills. I took them."

"No, you didn't. You put them in your pocket. I saw you."

"You saw nothing. I took my medicine."

"Show me. Empty your pocket."

"Okay, I put the pills in my pocket. I'll take them when I go upstairs."

"Take them now."

"You don't trust me."

"You just lied to me."

"Everybody lies sometime."

"That lie could kill you. If you don't take your medicine, you could have another stroke or a heart attack. Why do you do this to yourself? Why do you do this to me? I don't want you to die."

"Everybody dies sometime."

"True, but there is no reason to rush it. And there are worse things than dying. Do you want to have a massive stroke and end up still alive, but unable to think or talk or walk?"

"Everybody has a destiny."

"Is it your destiny to make things as hard as possible for me? Is it my destiny to do what I can to take care of you while you defy everything the doctor tells you to do?"

"Doctors don't know everything. Many times I don't take my medicine. I'm not dead yet."

"Nothing I say gets through to you, does it? Go to your sitting room and watch TV. Get out of my sight. I am so mad at you right now I can't think straight."

"Maybe you need medicine, not me."

"Dad, go! I need you to go before I say something I'll regret."

A Feeling You Wish You Didn't Have

The anger ebbed and flowed. The first time it hit me, right after Rodger returned home from an extensive stay in the hospital, I thought I was losing my mind.

I'd just spent months watching his mental health deteriorate as, unbeknownst to me, he'd been "cheeking" his daily antipsychotic meds, and spitting them into the toilet once he got out of my sight. His medication had been adjusted up, and then down; brands were changed and consultations scheduled over and over again.

Then it happened. One sunny Sunday afternoon, he lost his mind. Accusing me of trying to poison him, he ran down the street, moving at a pace that would normally be impossible for a man nearing eighty years old.

"She's trying to kill me!" He insisted, shaking with fear whenever I got too close.

He spent eight weeks in the psychiatric ward that time. Discharged on a Friday afternoon, he was back in the hospital Sunday evening. He had pneumonia. They

103

had sent him home sick. After a week in ICU, he was finally well enough to go into a medical ward. He'd also developed swallowing problems somewhere along the line. He had to have his food pureed, and his drinks thickened. He refused to eat slowly, and take small bites as the doctor ordered. As soon as his tray arrived, he'd grab a spoon and start shoveling the food into his mouth as fast as he could, and then he'd choke. So a nurse fed him each morning, and I made sure I was there for lunch and supper. Three weeks later, he was finally well enough to go home. Once there he seemed determined to start the dance all over again.

"I can take my medicine myself," he declared almost immediately upon returning home.

My anger reared its ugly head for the first time. I contemplated the downward spiral that would, inevitably, ensue if he were allowed to have his way.

I tried to pretend it wasn't there, but each time he tried to convince me to give him his pills, it grew stronger. I was royally ticked off that he would even try to manipulate me, again. I knew he would lie, and insist he was taking his medication when he wasn't. I was furious that he would subject me, and his son, to sleepless nights and hours of driving to and from the hospital to assure he received proper care. I resented that he seemed to think he was smarter than I was.

There were moments when I had to walk away as soon as he entered the room. I didn't even want to look at him. I was wracked with guilt, and questioned my basic humanity. How could I possibly be angry with this sick old man? The guilt was overwhelming. I prayed. I vented in the car when I went to the grocery store, and cried a lot.

I finally got some relief when I admitted my feelings to my husband. Mike assured me that it was normal to feel the way I did; that the job I'd taken on was harder than anyone could imagine, and what I was feeling is normal. I had nothing to feel guilty about. He took a couple of days off from work, and encouraged me to get out of the house.

"Go see a movie. Get a massage. Pamper yourself," he whispered. I cried on his shoulder. Relief mixed with the overwhelming sadness that I had, finally, allowed to engulf me.

ᘒ ✳ ᘓ

I couldn't concentrate on the movie. I spent the entire time in the theater trying to figure out what was wrong with me. I passed on the massage. I don't like strangers touching me. But I did go to the gym. An hour of aerobics helped ease the tension from my shoulders and neck. It felt good to sweat and push myself again. The next day, I went for a run on the treadmill. It was there that it all came together for me.

I wasn't just mad at him for trying to take control of his meds. I was mad at him for tricking us, and causing so much trouble. But I was *really* mad at him for not appreciating all I had done, and all I had been through. While I was busy caring for him, I'd lost my own mother to non Hodgkin's lymphoma. She was gone, and he was still here. She took all her treatments, and she died. He refused to do what he was supposed to do, and I got to nurse him back to health. It wasn't fair. He should be fighting with all he had just as she did. If anyone should still be here it should be...

In that moment, I heard a soft voice whisper... "It's not up to you to decide who lives." And then I heard a short, and very special phrase, that rings true no matter how often it's repeated. "Let go and let God."

I found myself nodding my head in agreement, and moments later, I began to feel better. I was able to go home refreshed, and take care of Dad again.

It wasn't a cure-all. The anger and resentment still came back sometimes when he was acting out. And I'd even gone so far as to tell God he had better get busy, as I'd let go a while ago, and he didn't seem to be doing anything to help. But finally, I recognized it for what it is.

>❊<

Rodger was doing the best he could with a mind that was failing in spite of all the love, and care, and medication, he was getting. And I was doing the best I could, in spite of all my weaknesses, and doubts. And God? He was there running alongside me on the treadmill, helping me get through the day.

LYNNE

The other day my friend, Sandy, asked me how taking care of Jack at home was going.

"It's the hardest thing I've ever done," I admitted. "There are times when I don't think I can go on. This man is the love of my life. We promised on our wedding day to be there for one another in sickness and in health. It was an easy promise to make when we were in our twenties with strong beautiful bodies and healthy minds. Sure, we knew we would age, but it was so far in the future it wasn't real. Our parents were old. Our grandparents were ancient. Growing old together was a romantic notion. I can assure you there is nothing romantic about being a fulltime caregiver. I am his wife. His lover. His partner. His is my rock. The one I turn to when life is hard, and I need someone to tell me everything will work out in the end.

At least that's the way it used to be. Now I am more nurse than wife. My lover is gone. I am in this alone, without my best friend. Most of the time I feel so alone I don't know where to turn.

"Then what do you do?" she asked.

"I remember all the good years we had. I remember the promise I made at the altar thirty-five years ago. I cry. And I pray."

"Does it help?" she said.

"Sometimes it does. On other days, I have to carry on anyway. What else can I do?"

Why Does It Have to Be So Hard?

I don't get it. Why is it so hard to do good work?"

"I don't know either, honey," my husband said. The creases in the corners of his beautiful brown eyes deepened, indicating he was trying to think of something to say that might help me with my struggle to understand why offering loving care to his father was always met with such resistance. He didn't come up with an answer that night, and neither did I. For weeks, I prayed and asked God the same question. *Why does it have to be so hard?*

I got my answer one Sunday morning. The priest began to speak after reading the gospel, and I felt he was talking directly to me.

"I've been hearing the same question over and over lately. 'Why is life so hard? Why is it so difficult to do good works?'"

A chill ran through me. God had heard my cry.

The priest lectured: "No one ever told you it was supposed to be easy. In fact there are many examples in the Bible of people being tested to their very limits. It's in adversity that you grow in spirit. It's when you step up and do the hard stuff God asks of you, that you earn your place in heaven. So quit whining, and do what you know has to be done, and remember you are not alone. He is there for you when you need Him."

After that, when things got very hard I tried to make light of it by telling Mike, "I earned my place in heaven today." He believed it, even when I didn't. I couldn't take the words of the priest to heart. I wanted a better answer. But, as things went on, and the more I repeated the words, "I earned my place in heaven today," the more at peace I felt. I was not alone. God was with me, and by doing the hard work, I was earning the grace to make it possible. Not easy. But easier. What I thought in moments of weakness and exhaustion to be impossible, became possible. Being a caregiver is not a job that we can do alone. We need help from our community, our family, and our friends. And in the moments when all of them are too busy, or too far away, there is One who is always there.

ALICE

I will not let my emotions get the best of me. I didn't get this far in life being weak. I'm the caregiver. I have no time for tears no matter how often they threaten. I bite my tongue, push them back, and carry on. Tears leave one depleted, exhausted, and wrung out. I don't have time for that. I'll cry when he is it peace. Only then, will I be able to let go. Until then, I will remain strong. I am the caregiver.

A Good Hard Cry

It had been brewing ever since my father-in-law's heart attack on Thanksgiving Day.

The day started off well with the sound of laughter resulting from the retelling of favorite family stories, and the scent of chocolate macadamia nut coffee and cinnamon toast filling the kitchen. Already the house was filling up with family. The counters were crowded with succulent dishes, lovingly prepped, and ready to be finished once the ham was done. The meat thermometer indicated the turkey was an hour away from perfection. Life was good and we were thankful.

At four the power went out. Still full of good cheer, and a glass or two of wine, I lit a fire in the fireplace, arranged a bunch of multi-hued candles in mismatched holders around the family room, and put the turkey on the grill. It all worked out. We had turkey, ham and stuffing by candlelight, and we not only would have leftovers the next day, we would have lots of freshly baked side dishes, too.

At 9:00 PM, we were in our car following the ambulance carrying Rodger to the nearest hospital to be stabilized, before he could be moved. Once at the new hospital he would receive an emergency catheterization, and have a stent inserted. He was in deep trouble, but he was getting swift, and proper care, and we were thankful.

A week later, he needed a pacemaker to keep him alive. He made it through that with relative ease. It didn't matter that his dementia worsened from the stress, and he spent much of his time deep in the past. Physically he was getting stronger every day, and who among us wouldn't want to go back in time to a farm in Italy on a warm summer day given the chance.

❧ ✻ ☙

Eleven days later, he came home, and we were thankful. He was weak and unsure what had happened to him. His memory was bad, and I was having a hard time getting his new medications adjusted. He developed swallowing problems, and a nurse needed to come twice a week. At night he raided the refrigerator, eating foods he wasn't supposed to have. He refused to wash until I filled a basin to bathe him. He couldn't be left alone, even for a few minutes. There went Christmas shopping—but he was alive, and we were thankful.

I was exhausted and I could feel the tears building behind my eyes. I wanted to cry all the time, but I didn't. I couldn't. I wasn't the weak one. I was the caregiver.

Then the phone rang. It was my stepbrother, my father was being rushed to a hospital in Florida. "Start praying," he said. "He has pneumonia, and a collapsed lung. At eighty-four, with lungs nearly destroyed by over fifty years of smoking, the doctor offers little hope he'll survive the emergency surgery he needs. I'll call you in an hour, or so, once he's out of surgery."

I prayed, and I prayed, and while I was doing that, I started packing for a trip that, I knew in my heart, would end with my father's funeral. And I waited for the call.

Two hours later, it came. When I heard my stepbrother's voice, I trembled, bracing myself for the worst. "He's okay. It's not pneumonia or a collapsed lung. Once the pulmonologist saw the x-rays, he canceled the surgery. Dad's dehydrated, and they have him on IV fluids. His vital signs are stabilizing. He's in the ICU for now, but he's going to be fine. I'll call you later with an update." With that, my stepbrother was gone.

❧❀☙

Stunned, I hit the end button on the phone, and put my head in my hands and cried. It wasn't a dainty cry with gentle tears moistening my cheek. It was a hard driving, gut wrenching, chest heaving, sloppy, ugly, sobbing cry. My nose ran, and my eyes burned from the force of it, and there were moments when I thought I might never stop. But I did. And then I started again. And again after that. And again after that, until my eyes were nearly swollen shut, and my head pounded, and my heart stopped aching.

I cried. I let it out. But you know what? That didn't make me weak. I was still the caregiver, and I was thankful. Both men survived, and I was thankful. And I was thankful for a good, hard cry.

CARRIE

I read a magazine article in the doctor's office the other day. I was waiting for Mom to have blood drawn for another test to determine if her blood is too thin. She's been on blood thinners ever since her heart attack. Anyway, the magazine article talked about a place that is combination day care center and nursing home. The pictures accompanying the piece showed adults beaming and reaching out to hug toddlers, who seemed to be enjoying all the attention. I wonder why no one thought of this before? No matter how tired, or out of sorts, Mom is, when my son brings his little boy to visit, Mom comes alive.

Great Grandma adores him, and he knows it, returning her devotion with as much love as his little body can hold. They communicate in a language only they can understand. It makes them both happy. I feel privileged to witness it.

As a young mother, I often longed for the day when my children would speak clearly, and my parents stopped offering so much advice. I was an adult, but I hadn't yet learned to appreciate the wisdom of a child, or the grace of old age. These two showed me both through their devotion to one another. I hope I am as lucky one day.

Big Turkey

From the first moment he saw her, Rodger was head over in heels in love with baby Ava. After the birth of my daughter's first child, he found out we would be going to their house each morning. He was up, and ready to go before sunrise every day.

"What time do we go?" he asked as soon as I wandered into the kitchen, and reached, bleary eyed, for a tea bag and my microwaveable cup.

"Not for a while yet. You have to have breakfast and take your medication. I need to take a shower, and get dressed. And besides, the new mom and dad need time to get going in the morning, too."

"They need us. We have to go."

Knowing he would pace, and worry until we got there, I sipped my tea on the way to my room, showered as fast as I could, and pulled on a sweat suit. My hair was hopeless. I put it in a pony tail, and grabbed a baseball cap to cover it. I packed a bag with his medications, a blood pressure monitor, thermometer, stethoscope, his nebulizer, band-aids, Depends, a change of clothes, and some food I knew he would eat. Just like I used to pack a diaper bag for my daughter when she was a baby. And now, she would do the same for her child.

As soon as we arrived, he went straight for the baby, who was nestled quite contentedly in the arms of her other grandmother.

"I'll hold her. I know what to do," he said, his tone of voice a clear indication he disapproved of her technique. Fortunately, my daughter's mother-in-law was amused rather than offended, and helped get baby, and great-grandfather, settled comfortably in the overstuffed chair he preferred.

And so it went. If the baby wasn't being fed or changed, he wanted to hold her, and he wasn't shy about chastising any of us for taking too long to hand her over. Often I would look over, and see her deep blue eyes staring into his faded brown ones, and thank God they had this time together. Was she transferring innocence to him as he silently shared his wisdom with her? I like to think so.

Lots of pictures were taken by proud parents and grandparents, of course.

One day, not long after our help was no longer needed, I gave Rodger one of the photos. In it, he was sitting in that overstuffed chair holding Ava, who was wrapped in a beautiful pink blanket. I knew he missed her, and waited to see him light up when he saw her. He stared at it for a few seconds, a puzzled look on his face, and said, "That's me."

"Yes, that's you." I answered.

He looked at it for another few seconds, before the smile I was hoping for, appeared. He tapped the picture, pointed to the baby, and announced, "Big Turkey. Happy Thanksgiving!"

♥❈♥

At the time, the proud new mama wasn't thrilled to think anyone could mistake her baby for a turkey. Now that years have passed, and Old Grampy, as Ava called him, is no longer with us, it's one of the most precious memories we have of him and the little girl he loved so much.

CYNTHIA

I know I'm not the patient, my brother, Robert, is. I know the doctor should talk with him, but it shouldn't stop there. I live with Robert. I take care of him, and I take him to every appointment. His dementia is advancing and the hallucinations and delusions are occurring more often. His years of schizophrenia add to the confusion, making it almost impossible to know which disease is causing his behavior on any given day. I wonder how much more his brain and body can take. Over fifty years of psychiatric care, hospital admissions, and powerful medications have taken a toll on both. His ability to reason is gone.

When he says he is not hearing voices the doctor nods in approval and tells me the medicine is working. I know better. I see the fear and panic in his eyes. I watch him spin and flap his arms for hours in his room. I'm the one who tries to calm him, and when that doesn't work I give him a sedative to allow him some peace.

Doctors ask the same questions every time. He tells them what they want to hear. Notes are typed into an electronic file and another appointment is scheduled. In a month we do it all again. If one more doctor tells me how lucky Robert is to have me, and then ignores my input, I am going to scream. Maybe then someone will listen. Or maybe I will be the one committed to the hospital.

Doctor, Do You Hear Me?

To a doctor schizophrenia is: "A long-term mental disorder of a type involving a breakdown in the relation between thought, emotion, and behavior, leading to faulty perception, inappropriate actions and feelings, withdrawal from reality and personal relationships into fantasy and delusion, and a sense of mental fragmentation." (Oxford dictionary definition of schizophrenia)

For his psychiatrist, the treatment for Rodger entailed medication to control his symptoms and regular visits to assess his thoughts and behavior. He was treating the disease. Every three months, Rodger would assure him he was taking his medication, and he was not experiencing hallucinations or hearing voices.

"She worries too much. Don't listen to her." They listened to him. They got tired of hearing from me.

At home I was dealing with the illness. Despite Rodger's insistence that everything was fine, I knew it was not. He paced the upstairs hall day and night, muttering and gesturing. I found him on his hands and knees trying to catch something scooting across the floor. Something only he could see. I reported all that, and more to his doctors on every visit.

I knew when he was hearing voices. It was evident in a certain tilt of his head as he listened to the silence around him. There were sudden bursts of laughter when he was alone in his room. The voices goaded him into seething resentment. I insisted he take his medicine. It resulted in accusations of mistreatment.

The doctors treated the disease the only way they knew how—more medication. It didn't work.

The others came, again, and again. Then they stayed. Relentless. Aggressive. Unyielding. He broke. His

117

mind a cyclone of confusion and suspicion. He arrived at the hospital in the back of police car.

"Why did you wait so long to bring him in?" the admitting doctor asked. "He is in desperate need of treatment." He called for an orderly to take Rodger to the psychiatric ward.

I'd been telling them for weeks. I was the one who worried. I was the one they should have listened to. Where they saw only the disease, I was living with the illness, and Rodger paid the price.

EMMA

I feel so alone, and yet, I am never by myself. Every day is the same. I wake up exhausted after spending the night responding to his bed alarm. He sleeps all day, and is awake and restless throughout the night. He has to pee. He can't pee because he woke me "to pee" two minutes ago. He wants something to eat. I bring him a snack only to take it away, he's not hungry. He's cold and I cover him with the blanket he kicked off a little while ago. It's too warm. I take it off and fold it at the foot of the bed for when he wants it again. This goes on for hours until it's time for his first C.O.P.D. breathing treatment of the day.

Once that is done, I wash him, and get him into clean pajamas. Next comes preparing his breakfast. It takes an hour to feed him. He resists taking small bites and swallowing three times to keep from choking and aspirating again. Another bout of pneumonia would be disastrous. Brushing his teeth is always an adventure. The worst is when he spits the saliva coated toothpaste out on me.

The rest of the day is more of the same. He demands. I respond. Not fast enough or in the right way for him—but I respond. Sometimes I think he hates me. Sometimes I begin to feel the same way about him.

Neither of us holds on to that feeling for very long. Somewhere inside, he knows I am his granddaughter. Somewhere inside, I know he is still the man who always made me laugh when he came to visit and I was a child. He taught me to play Jacks, and let me help plant the young tomato plants he put in each year, because he knew Grandma looked forward to them every summer. Even when he hates me, I love him, and I never could really hate him. I hate this disease.

When the visiting nurse asks how he feels, he says, "Fine." She looks at me, and I shrug. What's the use of saying anything else? Nothing ever changes.

FINE IS NOT THE ANSWER

How are things going with Rodger?"
"Fine."
"It must be hard."
"It's fine."
Are you taking care of yourself?"
"I'm fine."
"How is Mike dealing with all this?"
"He's fine."
"Do the two of you get any time away?"
"No, but we're fine."

So often when questioned by people, even the most well-meaning caregivers say they are fine. It's time to stop. FINE is not an answer. It's what we say when the person asking has no real interest in the answer, or has already proven that they are too busy, too disconnected, or too frightened to deal with what's happening.

Saying we are *fine* when we are not is a social norm that works most of the time. Why bore someone with details of our life when they are busy with their own problems? Aren't they asking about ours *only* to be polite?

How often do we greet friends or acquaintances with the words, "Hello, how are you?" Both parties know full well that we aren't asking for details, and the proper response is, "I'm fine. How are you?"

As a caregiver, I was guilty of saying it all the time. When I was so sleep deprived I could barely function, I carried on trying to convince everyone, including myself, that I was fine, and I'd sleep when the latest crisis had passed. When month after month of stress took a toll and triggered a panic attack, I breathed through it and went on. "I'm fine now," I'd say, once it was over. After a terrible argument with my husband, brought on by the same lack of sleep and a buildup of stress, we patched things up and promised not to let it get to us, again. We had a solid, loving marriage. We were simply going through a rough patch that would not last forever. We were fine.

Rodger was declining, and his need for care was increasing all the time. I was not taking care of myself, and the stress was taking a big toll on me. Mike was not fine no matter how hard he pretended he was. We needed time away, and would have given anything for someone to take over, even for one day.

Now I wonder what would have happened if I had responded truthfully.

"How are things going with Rodger?"

"Not good. He is getting weaker all the time. He hates being dependent, and it makes him angry. He takes it out on me."

"It must be hard."

"It's very hard. I'm isolated and lonely. I miss spending time with my friends and the people I used to work with."

"Are you taking care of yourself?

"There's no time for that. I had to cancel my last three doctor appointments to rush Rodger to the hospital when one of his illnesses worsened. Most days I eat on the run, and shower so fast I barely get wet, before I have to dry off and tend to his needs."

"How is Mike dealing with all this?"

"He is doing the best he can trying to be there for both Rodger and me, and still go to work every day. On the weekends he does all the shopping and runs all the errands that need to be done. He helps with Rodger in the evenings. There is no rest for him either."

"Do the two of you get any time away?

"No. We need a rest, but we don't know where to turn for help."

Would anyone have offered help, and a bit of respite, if I had not kept reassuring people that I was fine? I will never know, but I hope so.

KRISTIN

Dad was such a handsome man. The pictures of him the day he graduated from the Academy show him in his dress whites, tall and fit, his dark hair full and shining in the sun. His smile is the only thing that hasn't changed much. Sadly, it is rarely seen.

Some say I look like him, and there are moments when I see the resemblance. As I get older, more often, it's my mother's face I see in the mirror. She had her own quiet beauty, but even she admitted, Dad was the one people admired when they walked down the street hand in hand.

She's gone and he's fading more every day. The only thing colorful about him now is his language. Before he got sick he would never have talked like that. He took offence every time he heard someone using crude language, and called it cursing like a drunken sailor.

"A gentleman, even when he's had too much to drink, should have a better command of the language than that," he'd say.

Of course he knew those words, and probably said them when the occasion called for it, but never in mixed company. To speak like that to his only daughter would be unthinkable.

I can't repeat what he called me today. Not even on paper. Dementia is a hateful, obscene disease. I know a few words to better describe it, but my father taught me better than to use them. Sometimes I understand the people he used to chastise for cussing. At least once I'd like to forget about the extensive vocabulary he insisted I acquire, and curse a blue streak like they did then, and he does now. Wouldn't that be a moment to remember?

The Many Colors of Caregiving

Colorful is not the way one would typically describe the life of a caregiver, but once my father-in-law, Rodger, came to live with us my days began to revolve around the colors of his life.

Outwardly he appeared to be a drab little wren of a man. All his clothing was either brown or grey, the monotony broken only by one of the muted plaid shirts he saved to wear for an appointment with one of his many doctors. His lined, expressionless face would have been a blank canvas if not for deep brown eyes, topped by grey eyebrows, so overgrown, they rivaled those of the late Andy Rooney. When he spoke, there were no colorful sayings to add interest. "Just the facts, Ma'am." Everything about him seemed designed to blend into the background. Every day started, and ended, with a rainbow of colored pills, red, yellow, white, green, blue, and pink. Some were taken once a day, others two or three times a day, to treat or control his mental illness, Parkinson's disease, heart disease, Dysphagia, and various infections that seemed to pop up as often as weeds in summer. In between doses, billowing clouds of vapor from breathing treatments to ease his C.O.P.D. wafted out of his room. He counted out his various medications, and filled his pill box weekly, and he religiously inked in a mail order form when they began to run low. He knew when it was time for each pill, and never failed to take them on time. Or so it seemed.

I should have known what he was doing when the

symptoms first appeared, but I was still too green to know how devious he could be. Even his doctors were fooled until the day his mind shattered into shards of throbbing suspicion. As I write this, I try to imagine what a psychotic break looks like. I picture it as a swirling mass of colors so bright they burn his soul leaving him decimated, and his caregiver shrouded in deep, purple guilt.

Eventually I discovered that the anger and resentment I sometimes felt when dealing with the daily stress of life as a caregiver could hide in a fog of grey fatigue, or the flashing colors of an aura, signifying the onset of a migraine headache causing me to scramble to find what I could to minimize the pain.

Fortunately, not all the colors of caregiving are dark or somber. If they were, we couldn't do it. I treasured the bright blue moments of clarity, whenever they appeared. Like the day he told me how he and his brother, young men living in Italy, would roll up the carpets in the farmhouse kitchen in order to dance a tango with girls from the village. Was that a hint of pink pride on his face at the memory of holding a pretty woman in his arms? I basked in the bright yellow sunshine of joy when he gently held his newborn great granddaughter, Ava, for the first time, his eyes full of love for the tiny creature gazing up at him.

Yes, being a caregiver is a very colorful occupation. After Rodger passed away, and once the worst of the grieving eased, I realized that the moments we shared, the good and the not so good, would forever be part of the richly colored tapestry of stories being woven by caregivers who tend to their loved ones every day.

CARL

Dad could be so darn stubborn sometimes. His insistence that things be done his way often had me scratching my head trying to figure out how his brain worked. He had certain rituals that had to be followed. Any changes in his routine would result in a great deal of stress, pacing and mumbling that could last for hours. Whatever had gone wrong was due to some ongoing conspiracy to harm him. *They* were out to get him, and routine must be restored to keep *them* at bay.

Eventually I learned that trying to reason with him got us nowhere. In fact, it often made things worse. In his eyes, I had become one of the many unseen characters plotting against him.

As long as there wasn't possible danger to him, or others, I went along with him. Holidays were full of rituals. Christmas cards had to be displayed on the dining room table which would have been easy, except, they had to be in alphabetical order by first letter of the sender's last name. Imagine how many times the cards had to be rearranged. Is it any surprise that I hid some of them before he could see them?

St. Patrick's Day was another one that had me puzzled. Since we are not Irish, this day should have gone by without incident. Not for Dad, though. St. Patrick's Day meant not only wearing green, but eating green as well. I'm not talking a nice green salad or a portion of spinach, or lime Jell-O. Think more along the lines of the Dr. Seuss book, *Green Eggs and Ham*. I put food coloring in his scrambled eggs and boiled potatoes. Once I chopped some ham into small pieces and fried it with scallion greens and the dyed spuds. He picked out the ham. That got us through breakfast. Lunch was always asparagus and broccoli, dinner included Brussels sprouts, and avocado with kiwi for dessert.

The funny thing is, now that he's gone, I still display the Christmas cards on the dining room table alphabetically as he insisted, and I tuck some away for a few days before opening them, and adding them to the others. It seems right somehow. And I still celebrate St. Patrick's Day even though I'm not Irish.

Halloween Memories

"What time do the kids come?" My father-in-law asked that same question every year on Halloween.

"Six o'clock."

"Good. I eat at four. I'll have time to get ready."

I wondered what he had done to get ready before coming down from his room at precisely five forty-five. He looked no different than he had earlier. He'd be wearing the same brown flannel shirt tucked into brown pants, along with the black shoes and white sox he'd put on when he got up in the morning. He would have shaved that day, so his grey stubble wasn't as pronounced as the day before—but not because of the holiday. He shaved every three days, and had for years. His hair would be slicked back, as always, and his face would hold the same dour expression that greeted me every day.

"I hope I don't get too tired. I'm not as strong as I used to be."

"You don't have to give out the candy. I can do it," I said.

"No. I have to. It's my job," he insisted.

"Why? I did it before you came to live here. I can do it now if you want to stay in your room."

"I do it!" he snapped before moving a dining room chair close to the window and peering out to see if any ghosts or witches were coming.

Seeing the street was still clear of trick-or-treaters, he peered into the large wooden bowl full of candy, and started to mumble.

"I hope this is enough. She didn't buy enough. Oh, no."

"I have more. That's all that will fit in the bowl right now. I can add more as we need it."

"I can add more. It's up to me. What time do the kids come?"

"Six o'clock. If you get tired before they stop coming, let me know. I'll pass out the rest."

"I have to do it. I give them each one piece, right? What time do they come?"

"They should start coming at six o'clock. Give them more than one piece, we have plenty."

"Two pieces. I give them each two pieces. What time do they stop coming? I hope I don't get too tired. I'm not strong like I used to be."

"You don't have to do this. I can do it if it's too much for you."

"I told you, I have to do it. It's my job"

"Why?"

"Because I'm the oldest, and the oldest gives out the candy."

I didn't know what to say to that. In his mind that's the way it should be. Every year, as long as he was able, I let it him pass out the candy. I kept an eye on him, and when it was clear he was tiring, I made sure the bowl emptied, quickly turned out the light, and helped him back to his room. He always slept late the next morning, and woke proud that, once again, he had done his job.

Now I'm the oldest, and I give out the candy. I miss him.

DEANNA

There may not be light at the end of this tunnel, but there certainly is in his smile. I don't get to see it often, but when I do, I know the long sleepless nights and difficult days of confusion and anger are worth keeping him at home for as long as possible. I know there may come a time when I can no longer do this, not even with help. When it arrives, I will see to it that he is somewhere safe where he will get excellent care. I will visit as often as possible. We'll hold hands when we walk outside on warm days, and when the cold sets in we'll do the same as we walk the halls.

I always loved it when he reached for my hand in public. "Mine," he would say, and break into a smile full of love and mischief. "Mine," I would say back, pulling him a little closer.

Sometimes he does it when I'm sitting quietly next to him watching one of his favorite television programs. I feel a slight tug on my hand, look over, and there is that smile. "Mine," we say together.

Every day he smiles at me is another gift I cherish.

He Smiled Today

It didn't happen often. Rodger was a dour man with a deeply furrowed brow and a face rutted with frown lines. The landscape of his life, mapped out on the parchment-thin skin of the elderly, was a map of negative emotions. Fear, uncertainty, frustration, disappointment, and suspicion all left clearly marked passages across his countenance.

There were no laugh lines framing his mouth, or little crinkly fans of mirth around his eyes. A smile never came easy for him. Sometimes, when someone told a joke or shared a funny experience, I imagined his smile lying in wait, ready to spring out, if only he'd drop his guard for a moment.

The day it happened, I was there to see it. For a moment in time he forgot to worry, and ceased to contemplate all the things that didn't make sense. What brought this on, you ask? It was nothing, really.

The day started, as it always did, with his slow walk down the steps to the kitchen for his breakfast and morning medication. I took his vital signs, sent them off to the clinic for review via the tele-health monitor, and reassured him there was no bad news.

"Everything looks good." I smiled at him. "It's a good day to be happy."

"Yeah, happy," he grumped as he turned away.

"You look good this morning," I tried again.

"Looking is different than feeling," he insisted.

"Do you feel bad?" I asked, concerned that I'd missed something.

"No. I'm okay. That's it."

That's it, I thought. That's all there is for him. When there is nothing to worry about his slate is wiped clean. For a moment I felt like crying. He always looked so tired and sad. Then I remembered that he was fine, and it was a day to be grateful. I refused to let his funk engulf me.

"Don't worry, be happy," I sang out, loud enough to startle us both. As the off key words bounced off the walls, I started to giggle, and watched for some hint of mirth in him. But no, he continued up the stairs and shuffled into his room for a nap.

When 11:00 AM rolled around and he made his ever-so-punctual appearance for lunch, I expected more of the same. So as I sat across from him monitoring his intake and reminding him to swallow so as not to aspirate, I was surprised to see his lips moving. Is he talking to himself, I wondered, or responding to the voices that sometimes make it through the haze of medication designed to keep them silent?

And then I heard it, so soft and low I couldn't be sure it wasn't my imagination. I sat very still, and waited to see what would happen next. Before long he sensed that I was watching him, and slowly lifted his head, seemingly surprised to find me in my usual place.

"What's up?" he asked with all the disingenuous charm of a naughty three year old caught in an act of mischief.

"Are you singing?" I asked, nodding in approval.

"No, I don't sing," he answered gruffly. "But don't worry, be happy," he said with a big grin. And he blushed a delicate pink.

TRACEY

If I Don't Get a Sandwich Soon ...

G ive me some real food! If I don't get a sandwich soon I'm going to be a goner," my father-in-law, Rodger, demanded. Dysphagia had taken away his ability to swallow properly. He was frustrated, and angry, and taking it out on me.

"I'm going to tell the doctor. You wait and see. I'm going to tell him you're starving me to death."

I assured him that talking to the doctor was the right thing to do if he felt he was not being treated right. By the next office visit, he'd forgotten about the threat.

Despite feeling hurt by the accusation, my heart went out to him. I had to find a way to create meals that would bring him some measure of enjoyment, and maybe, in the process, ease his anger toward me.

For weeks I'd been preparing pureed food and thickened liquids. Neither one of which look very appetizing, nor do they satisfy the urge to chew. I showed him that the mushy stuff he insisted wasn't food was the same things he used to eat. I helped him mash the potatoes, prepare the vegetables, and put them in the food processor.

"This is real food," he finally admitted. *"But it's not as good. I need the real, real food."*

I wanted to serve him roast chicken, a baked potato, and fresh green beans with a slice of apple pie and ice cream for dessert. He should have been able to eat anything he wanted.

But the danger was too great.

I got creative. I pureed cupcakes with whipped cream and cherry juice on top to satisfy his sweet tooth. I made chicken stew with all the standard ingredients, and pureed it for him. The peas turned the stew green. It looked a bit odd, but it tasted good. I thickened nutritional drinks with bananas, peanut butter, and a bit of baby cereal to make milkshakes that didn't melt in his mouth. He loved them. I cooked with flavor and nutrition in mind.

Still the words, "If I don't get a sandwich soon I'm going be a goner," stuck with me. I lay awake at night trying to figure out how to make a sandwich that would be easy to swallow. Finally an idea came to me. I would puree a tuna sandwich.

Ingredients:

2 slices soft bread, crusts removed

1 small can light tuna in water, drained (white tuna not as easy to puree)

3-4 tablespoons of mayonnaise (add more if needed)

1 teaspoon of tomato juice

Milk

Directions:

Tear bread into pieces and place food processer.

Add two tablespoons of milk, puree until bread is a thick mush. (Add more as needed)

Divide pureed bread in half

Put tuna and mayonnaise in food processor and puree.

Place half the pureed bread on plate. Form it into a square to look like a sandwich slice.

Top with pureed tuna

Spoon tomato juice on top of tuna

Smooth remaining bread over top of tuna and tomato juice.

It wasn't perfect, but it helped him feel like he was finally getting a sandwich. That meant a lot to both of us.

Every day I tried to make him some version of the meal the rest of us were having. On Thanksgiving I put homemade gravy on pureed dressing, and mashed potatoes alongside organic turkey baby food. At the end of the meal he said, "This is just like my wife used to make." I knew it wasn't true, but as long as he enjoyed it, there was reason to be truly thankful.

MELANIE

I feel like I'm losing my mind. I finally got out of the house for an hour. It didn't matter that it was to go to the grocery store. It felt like a mini vacation to walk the aisles and look at the displays. To see people who don't need my attention. Even the awful piped in music sounded good to me as I selected things I wanted to buy. Gerry has been doing all the shopping while I take care of my dad. He's been doing all the other errands, too. I should be grateful, and most of the time I am. But sometimes I resent Gerry's freedom to come and go without worry.

Today I asked him to stay with Dad.

"I have to get out of here for a while or I am going to scream."

He understood and agreed right away. Grocery shopping shouldn't be considered recreation, but it was for me. I smiled at the cashier as I loaded my purchases onto the belt. I helped the bagger arrange the bags in my cart, and put my hand in my pocket to get my wallet. It wasn't there. In my rush to get out of the house, I'd left it sitting on the kitchen counter.

The cashier was very understanding. The person behind me in line was not. I began to panic and the store manager said everything would be okay. He took my cart to the office, and let me use his phone to call Gerry, who got our neighbor to stay with Dad, and he came to my rescue.

Once the bill was paid, I thanked the manager again for helping me.

"Don't worry about it. It happens sometimes with people your age." He smiled and patted my hand.

I wanted to tell him I'm not old, I'm exhausted, but I didn't. I was too tired to explain things. I just wanted to go home.

It's Not a Matter of Age

I knew when I arrived that it wasn't going to be easy to find a parking place. It was almost 11:00 AM, and the large lot usually fills up by 8:30 AM, and stays that way throughout the afternoon. I usually don't mind the walk. I'm healthy and enjoy not only the exercise, but the feel of the winter sun on my face. I have time to inhale the cool air before encountering all the antiseptic smells of the hospital.

I had my driver's license out, ready to present it to the guard as I pulled up to the gate. "Good morning," I greeted the woman on duty, fully expecting her to wave me through as she usually does.

"Ma'am, do you realize that the sticker on your license plate is expired?"

"Pardon me?" I didn't think I heard her right.

"Your registration is expired. I can't let you in."

For what seemed like ages I stared at her in disbelief. How could this have happened? We are usually meticulous with things like that.

My mind raced as I struggled to figure out how I could get to a meeting with Dad's doctors and the patient advocate, that I had called. The day before, someone had given him a razor and allowed him to shave on his own. A man with Parkinson's disease should never be given a standard razor, let alone, someone who was, also, taking four blood thinners. Put the two together and you end up with a face covered with tiny nicks and cuts that ooze for hours. Mike and I walked into Dad's room to find him looking as if he had been doing battle with Edward Scissorhands.

"What am I going to do?" I said out loud without realizing it.

"You can park at the 7/11 next door and walk in," the guard answered, taking pity on me.

And so I found myself walking across the wide grounds to the VA Hospital in Martinsburg, West Virginia in the rain. Fortunately, it wasn't too cold. Unfortunately, I was very tired from weeks of worrying about Dad, and long days spent at his bedside during this most recent crises. Still, I tried to convince myself that walking would be good for me.

What I hadn't figured on was that a rather short drive along the circuitous roadway becomes a baffling maze to one who has never tried it on foot.

As car after car passed me, I contemplated cutting across the lawns, but after one look at the soft ground and muddy patches between me and the hospital, decided it would be best to stay on the sidewalks.

It took me a while, but eventually I figured out how to get from point A to point B in time for the meeting without becoming completely soaked through. Everyone commiserated with my sad "expired tags" story before engaging in a very successful meeting, resulting in large signs posted in Dad's room. "NO RAZORS," read one in bright red letters. "THICKENED LIQUIDS ONLY, PLEASE," read another.

After the meeting, I visited with Dad for a couple of hours before starting on the return trek across the lots to the 7/11 to get my car.

"I hope I can find my way back," I muttered and raised my umbrella. Of course, I did, and the next day I arrived at the hospital with updated stickers on my license plates, and a renewed registration in the glove box.

VICKIE

"Too many cooks spoil the stew," they say. I say, "Too many healthcare professionals do more harm than good."

I'm old enough to have had a family doctor who knew and treated our whole family. He was there when I was born, and he was there when my grandmother passed away. He held her hand as she took her last breath, and he held my hand at her gravesite.

We didn't have to explain our family history each time we were sick. And at every visit he spent time talking to us, and really listening to what we had to say. I wish he were here now.

There would be no need for a team of doctors to see to Mom's care, none of whom know her. They rely on computer charts that are supposed to make it easier to access information and provide the whole picture. It doesn't work. Is it because they don't read what others enter in the chart? I think that's a big part of it. It's also because these wonderful programs are very much about billing, and less about personal care. Each procedure coded for accuracy.

When Mom had bronchitis and was admitted to the hospital, her dementia medication wasn't given to her. She wandered the halls trying to find a way out, insisting she had to get the kids ready for school. When she refused to eat, one doctor wanted to insert a feeding tube. Another said it wouldn't change the outcome for her, and it would cause her stress, and put her at risk for infection. How am I supposed to know who is right? Do they? What really concerns me is that each time a doctor sees her, there's a look at her chart before calling her by name, and before asking the same questions asked the time before. How can they know what's best for her? This isn't right. God, help us both.

You're Being Ridiculous

I couldn't believe I'd heard right. I had just gotten my father-in-law settled in a chair in the hospital dietician's office. We were there at the recommendation of the nurse assigned to him as part of the tele-health program.

Every morning I sent his blood pressure reading, pulse, temperature, and weight electronically to be reviewed by the nurse. If either of us saw a problem developing, we would contact the other, and decide how best to proceed. Rodger's hospital admissions had become fewer, and farther between, since he was approved for the program. I was grateful to have a partner when it came to dealing with his many doctors.

Both the nurse and I were monitoring his continuing weight loss. Every week he lost a pound or two. There was a time when that would have been a good thing. He'd had a tendency to be chubby, due in large part to the tasty food and large portions my late mother-in-law prepared for him. A typical Italian woman, food meant love to her, and anyone who sat at her table walked away well loved. But after several bouts of pneumonia, and a heart attack, he was in danger of losing too much. I was there to talk with an expert on how to enrich his intake without adding a lot of empty calories. I was stunned by her response.

"She worries too much," Rodger said, looking pleased while she lectured on about how I was overprotective and treating him like a baby. "I eat what I eat. That's it. Let's go home."

I wanted to respond as rudely as she had spoken to me. I wanted to walk out of her office and slam the door. I could feel my pulse quicken, and knew my face was flushed with color. Unfortunately, when one is blonde and pale skinned, it's almost impossible to hide anger or embarrassment. Both wash across my face in shades of pink to red depending on the situation. That day, I'm sure, I was glowing bright enough to light the entire room. But instead of blasting her, I took a deep breath. Then I pulled my chair up to her desk and took out the notebook I used to chart his vital signs each day. I knew they were in his hospital records, but I also knew that depending on where the information was stored in the file, it could easily be missed by the people who most needed to see it.

"Why would you say that?" I asked in a firm, but polite voice.

"His weight is within normal range. There is no need to be fussing over him."

"Hmm." I had to take a few seconds to gather my thoughts. The anger started to bubble up again. After all, I knew his needs, and his habits far better than she did. Why didn't she give me a chance to explain my concerns before judging me?

"I understand why it may appear that way. He is within normal range. My purpose for being here is so we can keep him there. Please, look at these figures. He is eating well, and he's losing two to three pounds a week. This has been going on for weeks. If he continues to lose at this rate he's going to be in trouble soon.

With a loud sigh of frustration, she took the notebook from me and began flipping the pages.

"I see what you mean," she finally admitted." But, he's still within normal weight. Don't get upset until there's a reason to get upset. You don't have to bring him in here for every little thing. And another thing, you walked in here with an attitude I didn't appreciate."

"And what was that?" I asked. "An attitude of concern for my father-in-law? Or was it the attitude of not taking your immediate insult and responding in kind? Perhaps it was my confidence in my ability to see a problem developing, and try to head it off, before disaster struck. In any case, I believe I'm done here. I'll figure this out myself."

I left knowing that Rodger was in better hands with me than with her, and I had behaved with more professionalism than she had. As we walked to the patient advocate's office, I did so with confidence and pride. When I reported her unseemly response to my request for help in solving a problem that could become life threatening, I was also being an advocate for the other caregivers that might walk through her door.

There was power in the knowledge that I knew best, and the attitude the dietician so resented was one that helped keep my loved one healthy.

It's important to know that not all hospital personnel appreciate or understand what we do as caregivers, or how precise our knowledge of the needs of those in our care can become. When you have to deal with one them, hold your ground and your temper, and do what you know is right. And make sure the patient advocate is aware of the problem. It may make things easier for the next caregiver in line.

VINCE

I had a dream last night. It scared the living crap out of me. In it, I was driving home from work at three o'clock in the morning. Not my usual habit, I assure you. The highway was eerily quiet. I drove for miles without seeing a single vehicle going in either direction. The sky was filled with clouds and hiding all but a sliver of moonlight. At first I enjoyed having the road to myself. No one hopping from lane to lane, no sudden stops as traffic backed up for any of the random reasons I'd come across on my normal commutes.

Then the radio came on by itself. I swear I didn't touch any of the dials on the dashboard. "Are you ready to die, Vince?" A sibilant voice filled the car.

Not believing what I heard, but creeped out enough to know I didn't want to hear the voice again, I turned the knob to off, and held my breath.

Silence.

Just as I became convinced the voice was all in my imagination, I heard it again.

"Are you ready to die, Vince?" This time the radio was off. The sound was in the air surrounding me.

"No!" I shouted. Cars apppeared, moving toward me at breakneck speed. One in each lane and an upcoming curve. There was nowhere to pull off the road, and I knew they were coming for me. My heart beat so fast and hard I could hear the beats echoing in my chest. Cold sweat poured off me. Seconds ticked by, and the cars continued to race toward me. Toward my death. I screamed in terror and the first slammed into my car.

The shriek of metal on metal and shattering glass announcing my doom, and then everything went black.

After what may have been minutes or hours I came to, the shriek of my alarm convinced me I was still very much alive. The sweat-soaked sheets were a testament to my previous fear. When I tried to get up, my legs buckled, weak from the intense emotion of the dreadful dream. I sat there, safe on my bed, wondering what was going on in my life to trigger a scenario like that. It was so vivid. My body and mind reacted to the stress as if it were really happening.

Is this what it's like for my brother when he's convinced there are people plotting to kill him? Does he feel terror like I felt when I was deep in my dream? I think I understand him better now.

What a cruel disease this is. Next time I won't try to convince him what he sees and feels isn't real. I will do everything I can to help him through it.

Normal Exaggerated

When I told you I was normal, I may have exaggerated slightly.

—Author Unknown

I love this thought. For people with Alzheimer's and other forms of dementia, their perception is reality. Their normal is different from ours. One moment Rodger would be living with his son and his pesky daughter-in-law, who insisted he use his walker, and made him eat pureed food when what he really wanted was pita bread, and a big juicy orange. "Pita bread is delicious you know." The next minute he had gone back in time. He was young, and strong, living on a farm in Italy. He had no idea who I was, or how I got in his house.

Sometimes he'd look up from the TV he watched hour after hour looking lost and confused. I always wondered where he was, and what he was seeing when that occurred.

He liked to watch reruns of old television shows. Bonanza was one of his favorites. He said it reminded him of Italy. When I asked him why, he looked puzzled for a moment before replying, "The way they cook all the time." I believe he was thinking of his mother, and how she would make polenta before going to church each morning and then come home to prepare meals for the rest of the day.

He loved to look at the Blue Ridge Mountains from the deck, or out the family room windows. "Those are hills," he insisted. "In Italy we have mountains."

The days when the voices came were hard for both of us. "They make me confused and suspicious," he told me. He would never tell anyone what they said to him. "Nothing good," his doctors told me. When I began to recognize the signs that he was hearing them I'd know "the others" were among us. I have to admit they made me suspicious too.

All this was part of his normal. It became a new normal for me as well. Normal was never knowing what would happen on any given day. Normal was accepting that things were not as they appeared to be most of the time. Saying that either one of us was normal was often more than a slight exaggeration.

SHARON

I'm trying to sleep, damn it. Go away. Get out of my head."
The earworm was relentless. *We Will Rock You*, by Queen of
all things, was stuck in my brain. I don't even like the song. I'd
heard it a million times when my son was a teenager. I cringed
each time the song ended only to be start again while he learned
to play it on his guitar. It didn't get stuck in my head then, so
why was it tormenting me now?

It had been a sixteen-hour day like so many others in the last
several months. The house was blessedly quiet. Dad was sleeping
soundly, for now, and I wanted desperately to do the same while
I had a chance. I was beginning to drowse when it started. I tried
thinking of other things, even silently singing other songs to
replace it. It simply would not stop. Hour after hour I tossed and
turned, and looked at the clock thinking ill thoughts about the
song and the band. I was getting desperate thinking I would be
awake all night again. I could not face another day like that. It
reminded me of the nights I lay awake worrying about my
children, and what the future would hold for them. Raising them
alone was the hardest thing I had ever done—until now.
Recalling how my son persevered in learning a new skill was
something I cherished, now. Perhaps that's what the song had
come to remind me. Life is hard, and more often than we would
like, it results in sleepless nights, but we can get through it. I just
hope if it happens again a different song gets stuck in my brain.

Please Make it Stop!

What time is it?"

"Eleven in the morning."

Thirty seconds later. "What time is it?"

Thinking he didn't hear me, I tell him again. "Eleven in the morning."

Thirty seconds later. "What time is it?"

I sigh, turn down the sound on the TV, and repeat the time once more.

Thirty seconds later. "What time is it?"

His mind was stuck in a loop. Before I understood what was happening, I would get frustrated and angry with him. He would go on like that for hours. Why did he do it? Didn't he know it was annoying as hell? I was convinced he did it on purpose in order to get attention, or to get back at me for controlling him as he often accused me of doing.

Then I learned more about dementia, and how the brain works. He wasn't doing it on purpose. He could no more stop repeating himself than a scratched old record album could stop from skipping when the needle reached a flawed groove. If you're too young to understand that reference, ask a baby boomer, he or she will explain it to you.

Once I understood what was happening, I figured out what to do. I had to move his thoughts past the flaw in the groove and then we could move on to the next section.

"What time is it?"

"It's almost time for lunch. Are you hungry?"

"No. What time is it?"

"It's time to wash your face. Here is a warm cloth."

The distraction helped for a few minutes, and then he asked again, "What time is it?"

"It's time to fold these towels. Will you help me?"

"Yes. I have to do something sometime. It's not good to sit and loaf all day."

A few minutes pass in blessed silence while he folds the towels, and I take them and unfold them, to keep him occupied.

And then it happened. He looked up from his work, and said, "My mother, she washed clothes on Monday. Monday was wash day." As he folded all the towels one more time, he began to relate another memory of his youth. The needle had moved on, and the result was truly music to my ears.

GAIL

I will never do this again. And I'm going to make sure my children never get stuck doing it either. I am going to see an attorney tomorrow, and do what needs to be done, now, to make sure there is enough money to cover my care in a nursing home or memory facility.

No child should have to bathe an elderly parent, wipe a bottom, or endure day, after day, mental abuse from a crazy person.

I know it's the disease. I've heard those words from medical professionals, the few friends I have left, and even my own family, but they don't live with it. I do.

I've been slapped, spit on, and called every foul name in the book for trying to help her. Who in their right mind would wish this on their children? Not me. You can count on that.

Was I Crazy?

You're a little bit crazy, you know that?" my father-in-law said.

It wasn't the first time he'd accused me of being crazy and it wasn't the last. Despite the fact that he'd suffered from mental illness long before age-related dementia set in, he was convinced he could take care of himself, and I was out of my mind to think otherwise.

Sometimes I agreed with him. About the crazy part anyway. Isn't it considered crazy to keep doing the same thing over and over expecting a different result? By that definition, we were both nuts.

He figured if he took every opportunity to take off down the hall without his walker when my back was turned, he'd convince everyone he didn't need it. After all, he'd only fallen once, and it didn't kill him. I hoped if I kept catching him, and leading him back to safety he'd begin to accept the walker, and use it without prompting.

When he developed dysphagia and could no longer swallow regular food and drink, I prepared fresh purees for him every day while doing everything I could to make them healthy and tasty. I learned that a lot of his favorite foods could be prepared that way. It was worth spending a bit of extra time so he could enjoy his own version of whatever meal we were having. Pureed hot dogs and potato salad on the 4th of July. Pureed turkey and dressing for Thanksgiving worked very well. So did the pureed pasta with homemade spaghetti sauce. I'm still proud of the pureed tuna and tomato sandwich and pureed cupcake he often had for lunch. Was I crazy to go to all that extra work instead of ordering prepared purees for him? There is a line of foods for people with dysphagia, and I did order some of them. But, I didn't want to rely on them. Eating was one of the few pleasures he had left, and I wanted him to experience the flavor of his favorites. He was convinced I was crazy to think food could be dangerous.

"Something's wrong with her. Food goes in your stomach not your lungs. You can't get pneumonia from eating," he'd tell the doctor at every visit. Eventually the doctors tuned him out, not bothering to explain, again, why he couldn't have a sandwich or big juicy orange.

Sometimes I couldn't help but wonder if I was crazy to become a caregiver. Was I crazy to lie awake at night trying to figure out new ways to get through to him?

Was I crazy to keep fighting for him, and with him, when it became clear that no matter what I did, or how hard I tried, he would continue to fail?

Maybe. But sometimes crazy is what it takes to get the job done. Maybe my crazy was just what his crazy needed at the time.

WESLEY

My mother died last month. I did what I could, but I couldn't save her. No one should have to go through what she did. I question why God would allow this to happen to a woman who never missed a Sunday mass. She prayed every day of her life. She never doubted God's presence in her life, even when things were hard. She thanked God for every blessing she received. She wasn't a saint, but she was as close to one as I will ever know. I will always miss her in this life and probably in the next, if there is one. I know I will not be joining her in heaven. Not when I failed her so badly. Not when I prayed for her passing so many times. Forgive me, Mom, I couldn't take it anymore.

The Agony of Relief

For seven years I was his constant companion. The one he railed against and accused of trying to poison him. The one he insisted was his best friend on the good days when he was lucid.

"Without her, I'd be a goner," he would say.

In the beginning, I was his chauffer taking him to his many doctor appointments. At first we took the forty-minute drive over the mountain to the VA hospital every three months. As his various ailments, including the dementia and Parkinson's disease, progressed the appointments came more often. Dysphagia came next. He could no longer swallow properly. His diet was limited to pureed food and thickened liquids. He had trouble swallowing his saliva. Aspiration pneumonia resulted in several long hospital stays and weakening him further, requiring doctor visits once a month. Then he had a heart attack, and a pacemaker was inserted. Blood clots developed in his arm as a result. Frequent blood tests to monitor his clotting ability and meant more trips to the hospital. Eventually we were going every week. He continued to fail, and eventually he entered home hospice care. We no longer made the drive.

He was hearing voices and became more delusional as the dementia progressed. The medication he had taken since his early twenties for schizophrenia began to lose effect. Still, we prayed for a miracle comeback. He'd done it before. We'd think we were losing him, prepare for the worst, and just when we began to lose hope, he would gather the inner resources and strength that had defined him all of his life.

He'd gone from farm boy to defiant resister of the Gestapo who had taken over his country. He moved to America as young man to start a new life. He enlisted in the Army to serve his new homeland. It was while in the service he had his first psychotic break. This brilliant man who spoke seven languages, and held advanced degrees in literature and mathematics would never be the same. Electric shock treatments, ice baths, experimental treatments and increasingly strong antipsychotic drugs robbed him of memory, and kept him sedated at all times. After thirteen years, he was released. He married and raised two sons. He was a hero in so many ways.

As he began to fail, I did too. Sleepless nights, constant stress, the guilt that came with knowing I couldn't save him, took its toll. The two of us were barely functioning.

I fed him. Changed his soiled clothing. Wiped his bottom. Bathed him. Dressed him. Sat up all night listening to him breathe. The night he died, Mike and I sat with him, holding his hand, and doing everything we could to keep him comfortable.

In the early hours of his eighty-third birthday, he took his last breath. This amazing man who had challenged me in so many ways, and taught me so much about what real strength of character looks like, was gone. It took a while for the tears to come.

"What's wrong with me?" I asked my husband.

And then it started. A slow trickle at first, followed by the first stabs of grief. I cried so long, I wondered if it would ever stop. When it finally did, I wiped my eyes, blew my nose and started over again, and again, and again. I cried until there were no more tears. It was only after I had exhausted my tears, and my body, that I could face the awful truth. It was not only grief that brought me to my knees. It was the agony of relief. His suffering was over, and that meant I was finally free. Intellectually I know my feelings were normal under the circumstances, but there is still a little voice inside that continues to ask, "What's wrong with me?"

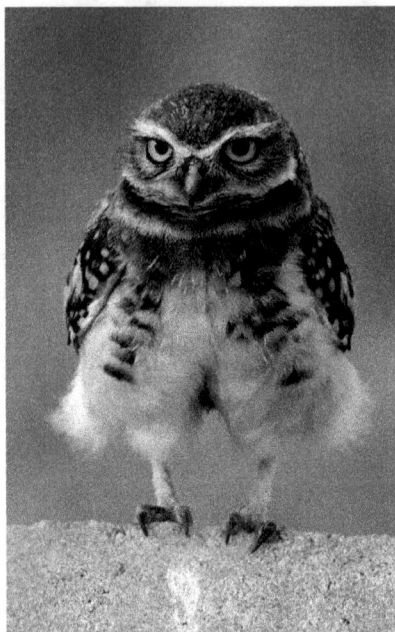

An Unexpected Visitor

When I see this funny looking little owl, I can't help but smile. It's as if Rodger has come to pay me a visit. With his stern face, pants riding too high, and arms firmly planted at his sides the little bird looks just like him. And just as it was when Rodger was here, I wonder what thoughts he finds impossible to express.

I believe our loved ones who have passed stay near and sometimes send us a reminder they are watching over us. That may be the case here, or it may be only my imagination. Either way it doesn't matter. I see him today and I am smiling.

THE END

About the Author

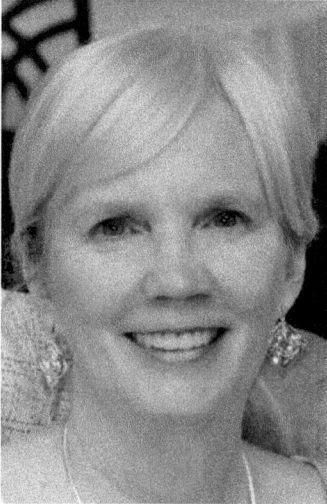

BOBBI CARDUCCI lives in Virginia with her husband, Michael. The years she cared for Rodger, described in her book, *Confessions of an Imperfect Caregiver* inspired a passion for caregiving. She learned how unprepared she was for the task, and how her lack of knowledge often impacted the one she was trying her best to help.

She wrote *You Are Not Alone* to help present and future care-givers learn more about what she calls "the hardest job you'll ever love."

Now a recognized speaker on caregiving issues, Bobbi's efforts to improve the lives of caregivers do not end with speaking and writing. She is a member of the Loudoun County Medical Reserve Corps, trained to assist members of her community in the case of catastrophic medical emergencies. She is on a team of people working to make Herndon, VA the first Dementia Friendly City in Virginia. *www.dfaherndon.org*

It is estimated that one in three seniors die with some form of dementia, and the numbers may double in the next ten to fifteen years. Bobbi developed a presentation designed to educate adults titled, *Prepare to Care: What Adults Need to Know About Alzheimer's/Dementia Before and After It Strikes Home.*

Bobbi's blog was chosen as a Top 50 Caregiver Blog in 2018. *www.theimperfectcaregiver.com*

Contact her through her website. *wwwbobbicarducci.com*

www.ingramcontent.com/pod-product-compliance
Lightning Source LLC
Chambersburg PA
CBHW060900280326
41934CB00007B/1124